ACCESS Health Press

# Live Longer

## What You Can Do, What Medicine Can Do

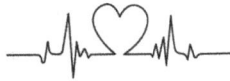

William A. Haseltine Ph.D.
And
Koloman Rath M.Ed.

# Acknowledgments

We thank the ACCESS Health U.S. team — Amara Thomas, Griffin McCombs, and Roberto Patarca — for their support in creating this book.

This work is supported by ACCESS Health International (www.accessh.org).

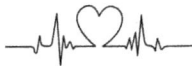

# Dedication

*William Haseltine, Ph.D.*

To my mentors and friends, you opened the road and were the wind behind me. Thank you for a wonderful life.

*Koloman Rath, M.Ed.*

To my parents, my siblings, and my loving partner — a building is only as solid as its foundation.

# Books by William A. Haseltine

Affordable Excellence: The Singapore Healthcare Story; William A Haseltine (2013)

Improving the Health of Mother and Child: Solutions from India; Priya Anant, Prabal Vikram Singh, Sofi Bergkvist, William A. Haseltine & Anita George (2014)

Modern Aging: A Practical Guide for Developers, Entrepreneurs, and Startups in the Silver Market; Edited by Sofia Widén, Stephanie Treschow, and William A. Haseltine (2015)

Aging with Dignity: Innovation and Challenge is Sweden-The Voice of Care Professionals; Sofia Widen and William A. Haseltine (2017)

Every Second Counts: Saving Two Million Lives. India's Emergency Response System.The EMRI Story; William A Haseltine (2017)

Voices in Dementia Care; Anna Dirksen and William A Haseltine (2018)

Aging Well; Jean Galiana and William A. Haseltine (2019)

World Class. Adversity, Transformation and Success and NYU Langone Health; William A. Haseltine (2019)

Science as a Superpower: My Lifelong Fight Against Disease And The Heroes Who Made It Possible; William A. Haseltine (2021)

The COVID-19 Textbook: Science, Medicine, and Public Health; William A. Haseltine and Roberto Pataraca (2023)

A Family Guide to Covid: Questions and Answers for Parents, Grandparents, and Children; William A. Haseltine (2020)

A Covid Back To School Guide: Questions and Answers for Parents and Students; William A. Haseltine (2020)

Covid Commentaries: A Chronicle of a Plague, Volumes I, II, III, IV, V, and VI; William A. Haseltine (2020)

My Lifelong Fight Against Disease: From Polio and AIDS to Covid-19; William A. Haseltine (2020)

Variants!: The Shape-Shifting Challenge of Covid-19 Vaccine Evasion & Reinfection; William A. Haseltine (2021)

Covid Related Post-traumatic Stress Disorder (CV-PTSD): What It Is And What To Do About It; William A. Haseltine (2021)

Natural Immunity And Covid-19: What It Is And How It Can Save Your Life; William A. Haseltine (2022)

Omicron: From Pandemic to Endemic; William A. Haseltine (2022)

Monoclonal Antibodies: The Once and Future Cure for Covid-19; William A. Haseltine and Griffin McCombs (2023)

The Future of Medicine: Healing Yourself: Regenerative Medicine Part One; William A. Haseltine (2023)

Viroids and Virusoids: Nature's Own mRNAs; William A. Haseltine and Koloman Rath (2023)

CAR T: A New Cure for Cancer, Autoimmune and Inherited Disease; William A. Haseltine and Amara Thomas (2023)

Ending Hepatitis C: A Seven-step Plan for a Successful Eradication Program: A Roadmap for Ending Endemic Disease Globally; William A. Haseltine and Kaelyn Varner (2023)

The COVID-19 Textbook: Science, Medicine and Public Health; William A. Haseltine and Roberto Patarca (2023)

Better Eyesight: What You and Modern Medicine Can Do to Improve Your Vision; William A. Haseltine and Kim Hazel (2024)

Molecular Biology of SARS-CoV-2: Opportunities for Antivirus Drug Development; William A. Haseltine and Roberto Patarca (2024)

Fusion! The Melding of Human and Machine Intelligence; William A. Haseltine and Griffin McCombs (2024)

# Contents

# INTRODUCTION
## The Pursuit of Longevity

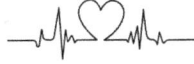

In the late nineties, I was invited to attend a conference in Como, Italy. The European Monetary Union's debut was fast approaching, and the event organizers decided to bring together a diverse group of movers and shakers to examine the implications. Former prime ministers and presidents, finance ministers, economists, philosophers, historians, novelists and journalists began to pour into the small, northern Italian city. A handful of business executives and scientists were also present.

On the second day, our host, the former (and future) Finance Minister of Italy, Giulio Tremonti, asked me to address the group before dinner that evening. I accepted, of course, but I wasn't sure what I wanted to discuss. Although a number of ideas were floating around in my head, I struggled to find the guiding thread that would pull them all together.

Midday gave way to afternoon, and afternoon to early evening. While mulling over what to say, I paced the gardens of the conference hotel, the charming Villa d'Este on the shores of Lake Como. It was on the cusp of fall, and a crisp breeze cut through the air. I paused for a moment, distracted by the dying rays of the evening sun as they lit up the surrounding mountains. Soon, the leaves would begin to drop, followed not long after by blankets of snow. And still, the mountains would stand tall. Compared to these stoic rock giants, isn't life painfully fragile? I will be gone, but the mountains will remain.

In that instant, I was jolted by a concept so contradictory it registered almost like a physical blow: I had it all backwards!

It is life that endures, not mountains. Go back many millions of years, and the gorgeous peaks of the Pre-Alps are nowhere to be seen. Skip forward many millions, and again, they may be gone. But what has been present throughout is *life*. All life is united by an immortal molecule, DNA, that has existed for billions of years. Yes, it takes different forms, but all are variants of the original. One parent molecule divides and gives rise to two almost identical daughters. Both are originals. The immortal molecule continues its journey from the unimaginably distant past. We —all forms of life— are but its carriers, pausing briefly along the way.

I knew I had found the leitmotif for my talk. And even now, all these years later, the power of that realization has not lessened its grip on me. In fact, it is what spurred me to write this book that you are currently taking the time to read.

~●

But notice, there's a frustrating paradox at play: while DNA, the molecule that underlies all life, has persisted for eons, you and I, and almost every other living being, have a finite expiration date. What if we could slowly close the gap between the permanence of DNA, on the one hand, and our very real mortality on the other? Might we be able to link our individual existence to the fundamental immortality of life?

The first step of any solution is knowing where to look. And what better place to look for role models than trees, many of which are notoriously long-lived. Indeed, the world's oldest recorded tree was a Great Basin bristlecone pine dubbed "Prometheus," which was close to 5,000 years old at the time it was, tragically, cut down in 1967. The second-oldest tree we know of, another bristlecone pine, and this one still living, is playing catch-up and quickly approaching 4,900 years of age. For these steadfast survivors, decades must feel like mere months.

Trees possess another ingenious feature that grants them a kind of quasi-immortality: the ability to regenerate. Take a tree, cut off a branch, stick it in the ground and start watering it. Slowly, it will begin to grow into a full-blown tree. Granted, it's hard to judge whether we should consider this "derivative" tree an extension of the original or a new being in its own right.

We can take it one step further. There's a jellyfish, *Turritopsis dohrnii*, that can live forever. Any time it sustains an injury, or even the threat of starvation, this creature "reverse ages." Its cells undergo a process known as transdifferentiation, which is when one type of cell turns into a completely different type of cell, allowing the jellyfish to metamorphose back into a juvenile stage of its development. From here, it can begin again from square one. To draw a parallel, it's as if we could revert back into our baby selves any time we felt endangered by disease, injury, or plain old age.

These jellyfish exhibit what scientists call "biological immortality." Make no mistake, they can still die — predators remain a threat, as does extreme physical damage — but their risk of death does not increase as they age. In practice, this means they have managed to uncouple chronological age from the aging process. While we become frail with age, and the risk of mortality increases accordingly, these animals do not. They are eternally young.

Of course, leaping back into a juvenile state is not exactly what we think of when we talk of longevity; we don't want to lose all of the memories we've gathered over the years, the very memories, it could be argued, that make us who we are. What good is "immortality" if we have to give up our sense of self every time we revert to a youthful state?

Regardless, the exceptional longevity of the aforementioned organisms acts as a substantial "proof of principle": *there is no lifespan inherent in DNA* — the molecule itself is immortal *as long as* it maintains its integrity and the integrity of the genes it encodes for. Easier said than done. But what if there were a way of resetting DNA to square one, of getting rid of all its accumulated wear and tear?

Nature does provide us with a preliminary blueprint. Think about it, any time a living creature reproduces, it creates something new from something old; it is concocting youth from age. For example, a man in his seventies and a woman in her late thirties may decide to have a child. Despite their own advanced combined age, they can come together to give life to a newborn infant. The clock of time ticks steadily on within each of us, and yet, it is reset to almost zero every time a child is born.

We know that at the heart of each cell lies DNA, the molecule that carries the instructions to build our body. It is this same DNA that is rejuvenated when an egg is fertilized by a sperm — the aged DNA is reverted to its original form.

Although magical, this doesn't address the issue of our *individual* mortality. Sure, at the species level, we can reset the aging clock through reproduction, but at the individual level, we don't have this power. It's as if it has been compartmentalized, only drawn upon for reproduction.

During the speech I gave in Italy in 1999, I speculated that something about the environment of the egg must help reset old DNA back to its primal state. If we could harness these signals, I thought, we might be able to convert aged cells back to a youthful state.

I would have to wait until 2006 for my predictions to come true, when Shinya Yamanaka discovered the key genes active in the fertilized egg that rewind the biological clock; these genes are so powerful that they return even highly specialized adult cells, skin cells, for example, to the equivalent of a fertilized ovum. Yamanaka called these cells *induced pluripotent stem cells*, or iPS cells, for short.

And isn't that what we really expect from modern medicine? We yearn for it to bring our bodies back to their healthy state, whether they've been damaged by injury, weakened by disease, or weathered by time. While preparing my speech, I realized that we needed a word for this new form of medicine — one that doesn't just fix, but renews and rejuvenates. It was then that I coined the term *regenerative medicine*.

The above ideas may ring of science fiction to you, but if the past hundred years of medical and technological advances have taught us anything, it is that science fiction is often just a few steps ahead of the game; what starts as a far-fetched idea in some book becomes reality a number of decades later. I don't expect it to be any different in this case, especially considering every single one of us has skin in the game: who doesn't want to live a longer, healthier life?

You only need to look as far as the pyramids in Egypt or the mythical fountain of youth to realize that the dream of eternal life has been with us since the beginning. To be mortal is to wish to be immortal. And now, with the guiding hand of science, we may be on our way to making our shared dream a reality.

By investigating how we age, or, put differently, *how we die*, we can slowly piece together the longevity puzzle. By identifying the principles that govern the aging process, we can glean an understanding of where we might be able to intervene.

Intervention, however, doesn't just mean extending lifespan. Although that's the most obvious metric by which to gauge our progress, it is not the only one. After all, what good is a longer life if more of it is spent in ill-health and frailty? What we really want — and should be striving for— is not just longer life, but healthier life. We want to be able to do the things we love, for longer. We want to be able to play our favorite instruments, or go for a run, or spend time with friends and family. Simply tacking on additional years of life devoid of the things that make life worthwhile doesn't seem especially enticing. So, the goal is actually twofold: first, learn to extend health into old age, and second, extend lifespan.

While we're fighting an uphill battle, I am convinced that patient, sustained research will allow us to crack the longevity code. But we also need to keep a level head; snake-oil salesmen thrive in times of uncertainty, and a field with stakes as high as this one is bound to attract them in droves. By giving you a solid overview of the principles of aging, I hope this book will help bolster your understanding and equip you with the knowledge needed to separate the hype from the science.

# PART I

# What is Aging?

# CHAPTER 1

# The "Why" and "What" of Aging

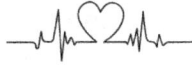

When it comes to aging, two questions jump out: *why* and *what?* Though it may seem like a strange claim, it's not obvious that we *need* to age. Like the jellyfish I mentioned earlier, it's possible to imagine a decoupling between chronological age — the number of birthdays you've celebrated — and the risk of disease and death. So, *why* is it that as we grow older we also begin to decline in health and vitality? And to follow up on this, *what* exactly *is* aging?

## Why Do We Age?

Let's tackle the 'why' first. In 1957, the American biologist George C. Williams proposed an elegantly simple evolutionary explanation: certain genes, he suggested, could have dual effects: they may be beneficial early in life and detrimental later on. Essentially, these genes provide advantages for survival and reproduction during youth but come with a cost as we age.

To make sense of this theory, you have to realize that natural selection is all about passing on genes to the next generation. It favors traits that enhance an organism's ability to survive and reproduce. If a gene helps you stay strong, healthy, and fertile during your reproductive years, it's likely to be favored by evolution, even if that same gene causes problems later in life when you're past your reproductive prime.

Williams' theory also explains why these genes haven't been eliminated over the span of human existence: in the eyes of evolution, they simply aren't harmful (even if now, from the comforts of modern life, we've come to hold a grudge against them). Natural selection "favors" traits that boost reproductive success, meaning it overlooks the negative impacts that manifest only in old age, after the prime reproductive period has passed. This evolutionary trade-off means that our bodies are optimized for the propagation of our genes, not necessarily for long-term health.

While this continues to be the dominant theory for the origins of aging, it is not without its critics. This shouldn't be surprising — there is rarely full consensus on any topic in science. But for now, it's the best answer we have.

Still, it doesn't provide a full account of the situation. For example, it doesn't really tell us why different animals age at different rates. Consider for a moment the natural variability in lifespans found across the animal kingdom. Some creatures, like mice and hummingbirds, live only a handful of years. Mayflies, only a number of hours. While others, I'm thinking of the Greenland shark and the Galapagos tortoise, can live hundreds of years.

A key to this puzzle lies in the concept of "live fast, die young." Species that live in environments with high predation risk or limited resources tend to prioritize rapid growth and reproduction, often at the expense of long-term maintenance and repair. Their metabolic engines burn fast, favoring immediate survival over longevity.

This strategy makes sense in an evolutionary context. For animals like mice, which face a constant threat of predation, investing energy in building long-lasting cellular structures or robust repair mechanisms would be futile — most won't live long enough to benefit. Instead, these animals channel resources into reproducing as quickly as possible, ensuring their genes persist even if their individual lives are cut short. In contrast, species like tortoises or whales, which occupy relatively low-risk ecological niches, can afford to invest in cellular maintenance and repair, extending their lifespans.

While metabolism and energy trade-offs provide valuable insights into aging, the two alone don't fully explain why some species age faster than others. The missing link may be something called "biosynthetic cost" — the energy required to produce high-quality biological materials. This includes the process of assembling proteins, ensuring their quality, and replacing faulty components. Essentially, species that invest more energy into producing durable, error-free biological structures tend to age more slowly and live longer lives.

Take the example of the naked mole rat versus the mouse. Although they are of similar size, the naked mole rat has a biosynthetic cost over three times higher than that of a mouse. This means it spends significantly more energy ensuring that its proteins are of high quality, which in turn makes its tissues more resilient to stress and damage. The result? Naked mole rats can live up to 30 years, while mice typically survive only two to three years. The mouse, by contrast, grows rapidly and reproduces quickly, prioritizing speed over quality — a trade-off that leads to shorter lifespans.

Intuitively, this makes sense. A house with a solid foundation will be more resilient and sturdy than one that has been rushed. Or even more simply: things of good quality tend to last longer. There's a reason dollar-store goods are cheap!

This same principle appears to apply to us — living, breathing animals. Those that develop more quickly are more likely to attain reproductive maturity compared to those that grow at a slower pace; however, this rapid growth comes at the cost of producing lower-quality biomaterials. Life expectancy drops accordingly, and so does the chance of reproducing later in life (an option that remains available to those that evolve slowly and steadily).

## Well, *What* Is It?

That leaves the 'what' of aging. Unfortunately, consensus is even harder to come by when trying to answer this one. In 2022, Vadim Gladyshev, a gerontology researcher based at Harvard Medical School, surveyed 100 of his colleagues at a conference on aging. He quickly realized that there is very little agreement about, well, anything. Asked to explain what aging is, roughly a third-of respondents defined it as a gradual loss of function — the "wear and tear" of daily life leads to a deterioration of cells and tissues in the body over time, similar to how mechanical parts in a machine deteriorate with usage. Others favor a different approach, suggesting that aging is less about wear and more about the accumulation of molecular gunk and DNA lesions, known as "deleterious changes." Another stance defined aging along purely demographic lines, stating that it is simply an increase in the chance of dying.

Asking whether aging is a disease or not led to a similar difference of opinion: while more than a third of those surveyed agreed that it is, 38% thought that it isn't. The remaining 28% were undecided. Some even flipped the question on its head, asking if many diseases couldn't actually be considered as accelerated aging in specific organs or systems of the body.

Even *when* aging starts is up for grabs, albeit most experts fall into one of four categories: those who consider aging to begin before conception (the older your parents at conception, the further you are in your aging process), those who consider aging to begin at birth, those who think it starts at puberty, and those who say it doesn't start until we stop developing (early adulthood).

And new findings, hot off the press, further complicate the picture. Although the above stances disagree about *when* we start to age, they all implicitly agree that, once we do, it's a steady onward march. This may not be so. Recent data suggest that, instead of following a linear path, our aging journey may actually progress along peaks and plateaus; extended periods of minor aging followed by sharp spikes during which we age rapidly. These spikes are marked by significant changes in the composition and behavior of cell populations within the body. Adding to the puzzle, these "aging milestones" are not evenly spaced. One of the more noticeable spikes happens in our mid forties, while another strikes in our early sixties. While surprising, and deeply unintuitive, this "topographic" view of aging may soon become the established paradigm.

Taken at face value, the depth of disagreement around the nature of aging might come across as quite discouraging; if we can't even agree on what it is, how are we ever supposed to do anything about it? But you might also consider it a mark of opportunity. The conflicting views are just a manifestation of the many unknowns still to be addressed. This isn't something we should despair about; it's something we should look forward to. What we currently know and can do about aging is just the beginning — so many exciting discoveries still lie ahead of us. What would be really frightening is if we already knew everything there was to know about aging *and still* had no way of fighting back against it.

# CHAPTER 2

# The Hallmarks of Aging

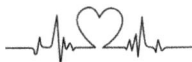

—∿∿♡2∿∿—

As part of the journey to track down the sources of aging, we need to distinguish between "driver" and "passenger" mechanisms. Drivers are the "root causes" of aging, while passengers are the byproducts of these underlying processes.

This distinction is essential. Mistaking the symptoms of aging as the causes would be akin to mistaking the blood pooling around an open wound as the cause of the injury itself. Or, to keep things on topic, it would be like assuming that gray hair, which is a visible marker of getting older, is actually the reason we age in the first place. Of course, we understand that's not how it works; it is simply a passenger, a sign of what is happening underneath. But untangling the arrows of causation isn't always that easy, especially once you move into the realm of biomolecules.

So, where *should* we look for answers? In 2013, a pivotal paper spearheaded by Spanish scientist Carlos Lopez-Otin outlined nine core mechanisms that work together — or sometimes against each other — to drive the aging process. He and his colleagues decided to call these mechanisms "the hallmarks of aging." Thus was born a unifying framework to help make sense of the biological forces behind aging.

To qualify as a "hallmark," each process had to meet three criteria. It had to show up during normal aging, be experimentally tweakable to speed up aging, and, perhaps most importantly, be reversible —

at least in theory. This final criterion was crucial because it hinted at the possibility of improving years spent in good health, or extending life altogether, by targeting these mechanisms. The framework has quickly become a cornerstone of aging research, helping researchers link diverse studies under a unified concept.

In 2023, the framework expanded to include three new hallmarks, reflecting how much our understanding of aging has grown over the past decade. These additions addressed gaps in the original framework, drawing attention to processes like the breakdown of cellular waste-clearing systems, disruptions in how cells sense nutrients, and the miscommunication between cells that becomes more common with age. Together, these updates capture the increasingly complex picture of aging as a biological phenomenon that operates on multiple levels, from molecular machinery to whole-body systems.

Before we launch into the hallmarks themselves, I should mention that they can be broken down into three categories: primary, antagonistic, and integrative. The primary hallmarks are those that we can say, with a fair amount of confidence, directly drive cellular damage. They are the most blatant "causes" of aging: DNA damage, telomere shortening, epigenetic alterations, loss of proteostasis, and disabled macroautophagy.

The next group, so-called antagonistic hallmarks, are in conversation with the primary hallmarks; they kick off in response to initial damage, with the goal of fixing the issue. In small doses, they are beneficial. But you can have too much of a good thing, and the intensity of the response can reach a tipping point where it slides from helpful to harmful. This group includes: deregulated nutrient sensing, mitochondrial dysfunction, and cellular senescence.

Finally, the integrative hallmarks emerge once the accumulated damage of the other two groups is so severe that cells can no longer maintain their usual internal balance. This leads to a breakdown in cells' repair and maintenance processes, pushing cellular damage past a point of no return. Think of these hallmarks as the final blow in a multi-punch knockout combo. This group includes: stem cell exhaustion, altered intercellular communication, chronic inflammation, and dysbiosis.

I should also mention that these same hallmarks will pop up time and again throughout the book, including in later chapters where I discuss the way lifestyle decisions influence longevity and how recent medical advances might, down the road, help us live longer lives. All that to say, *nota bene.*

# CHAPTER 3

# DNA Damage: A Silent Driver of Aging

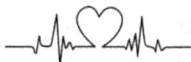

A mong the most promising candidates for a driver mechanism of aging is DNA damage — a subtle but relentless process that deteriorates the body from within.

DNA, the molecule that encodes the genetic blueprint for all life, is constantly under attack. Every day, each cell in the human body experiences tens of thousands of lesions: tiny breaks, mutations, and errors that can throw the cell's processes into disarray. These lesions come in several forms. Single-strand breaks are relatively minor, affecting just one side of the DNA double helix, but double-strand breaks — where both sides of the DNA ladder are severed — are catastrophic. Other types of damage include mismatches during DNA replication, in which the wrong genetic "letter" is inserted, potentially causing downstream errors that accumulate over time.

As our bodies age, the ability to repair DNA becomes less efficient, and mutations build up. This accumulation leads to widespread cellular dysfunction and contributes to many of the diseases we associate with aging, from cancer to neurodegeneration. The primary sources of DNA damage are both external and internal. Ultraviolet (UV) radiation from the sun, smoking, pollution, and exposure to certain chemicals can all break or mutate DNA. However, much of the damage is self-inflicted — a byproduct of essential cellular processes that keep us alive.

Cells can repair some DNA damage effectively through various mechanisms such as base excision repair, nucleotide excision repair, and mismatch repair. However, as we age, these mechanisms slow down, allowing damage to accumulate. Single-strand breaks can generally be patched up, but double-strand breaks present a much bigger challenge. The more these errors build up, the more likely it is for cells to enter a state of senescence (permanent arrest) or, worse, become cancerous.

~~●

## Oxidative Stress: The Fire Within

One of the most significant internal sources of DNA damage is oxidative stress. This process occurs when there's an imbalance between free radicals — unstable, reactive molecules — and the antioxidants that neutralize them. Free radicals are created as a natural consequence of metabolism, the process through which cells produce energy. If metabolism is like a controlled fire burning within each cell, free radicals are the sparks that fly off that fire. In small amounts, they are useful, playing essential roles in immune response and cell signaling. But when they accumulate unchecked, they can wreak havoc.

Oxidative stress is particularly dangerous because it can damage not just DNA but also proteins and cell membranes. The free radicals generated during metabolism can strike DNA, breaking its strands or causing mutations. Over time, the body's ability to neutralize these molecules declines. Factors like smoking, excessive alcohol consumption, poor diet, and environmental toxins can all exacerbate oxidative stress, accelerating the DNA damage that contributes to aging. Even chronic psychological stress and poor sleep have been linked to increased oxidative stress, tipping the balance further in favor of free radicals.

At the molecular level, free radicals are unstable because they have an unpaired electron. This makes them highly reactive, as they seek to "steal" electrons from nearby molecules, including DNA, proteins, and lipids. This electron theft can break chemical bonds or create new ones, resulting in the destabilization of the affected molecules. In DNA, oxidative damage can lead to base modifications, strand breaks, and even cross-linking between DNA and proteins, further disrupting cellular function. Antioxidants — such as vitamins C and E, selenium, and glutathione — are the body's natural defense, neutralizing free radicals by donating electrons without becoming reactive themselves.

~✎

## Lessons from Nature

Humans are far from the only species that deal with the challenge of DNA damage and repair. Some animals have evolved remarkable strategies to combat the accumulation of damage, allowing them to live far longer, healthier lives than would be expected for their size or environment. Two of the most fascinating examples are the naked mole-rat and the bowhead whale.

The naked mole-rat, a small, wrinkled rodent that lives in underground colonies in East Africa, is famous for its longevity and resistance to cancer. Whereas most rodents live just a few years, the naked mole-rat can live over 30 years. One of the key factors behind its extraordinary lifespan is its ability to resist DNA damage. Studies have shown that naked mole-rats have more efficient DNA repair mechanisms than humans, particularly when it comes to fixing double-strand breaks — the most dangerous type of DNA lesion. Their cells also produce high levels of a protective protein called HSP70, which helps maintain protein stability and assists in the repair of damaged DNA.

In addition to their superior DNA repair abilities, naked mole-rats produce fewer free radicals than other animals their size, which limits oxidative damage to their DNA. The combination of reduced oxidative stress and efficient DNA repair allows them to maintain cellular integrity far longer than most other mammals. Research suggests that their cells have an enhanced ability to detect DNA damage early, allowing them to activate repair mechanisms before the damage becomes too severe.

Even more impressive is the bowhead whale, a giant of the Arctic that can live over 200 years. Bowhead whales are one of the longest-living mammals on Earth, largely due to their exceptional DNA repair mechanisms. Their cells have been shown to repair damage more accurately than those of shorter-lived species, likely contributing to their remarkable longevity. One of the most intriguing discoveries about the bowhead whale is that it has multiple copies of a gene involved in DNA repair, offering extra redundancy in the case of damage. This genetic duplication may give bowhead whales an edge in repairing the kinds of mutations that accumulate over time in other species.

Compared to humans, both the naked mole-rat and the bowhead whale have evolved enhanced DNA repair capabilities that not only protect them from age-related diseases but also allow them to live longer without the cellular decline that typically accompanies aging.

~~~

## The Toughest Survivor: Deinococcus Radiodurans

If we're talking about champions of DNA repair, no organism is more remarkable than *Deinococcus radiodurans*, often called "the toughest bacterium in the world." This microbe, discovered in the 1950s, has the extraordinary ability to survive in environments that would destroy most forms of life, including areas exposed to nuclear radiation.

While humans begin to suffer health consequences from radiation exposure at around 100 millisieverts (mSv), and a dose of 5,000 mSv is lethal, *Deinococcus radiodurans* can survive exposure to 15,000 grays — 5,000 times the dose that would kill a human. How does it manage this feat? Its DNA may shatter into hundreds of pieces upon exposure to high levels of radiation, but within hours, the bacterium's repair mechanisms go to work, piecing its genome back together with remarkable precision.

One of the secrets to *Deinococcus radiodurans'* success is its redundant genome — it has multiple copies of its DNA, which provides templates for accurate repair. It also produces a range of proteins that help stabilize broken DNA and facilitate its repair. In addition, the bacterium has an efficient system for clearing away free radicals, which means that oxidative stress, a major driver of DNA damage in other organisms, poses little threat to it.

Although humans can't hope to mimic the resilience of *Deinococcus radiodurans*, studying how this microbe repairs its

DNA so effectively may offer insights into improving human DNA repair mechanisms. If we can learn to harness even a fraction of its repair capabilities, we may one day be able to slow the aging process and reduce the risk of age-related diseases.

# CHAPTER 4

# Telomere Attrition: The Fraying Ends of Youth

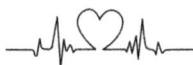

—ⅉⅉ♡ⅉⅉ—

Imagine your chromosomes as long, delicate shoelaces, and at each end of those shoelaces are telomeres — protective caps that prevent the chromosomes from fraying. Much like how the plastic tips on shoelaces protect them from unraveling, telomeres guard our genetic material, ensuring that every time a cell divides, the entire chromosome remains intact. However, with each round of cell division, these telomeres shorten. Eventually, they become so short that they can no longer protect the chromosomes, causing the cell to stop dividing or causing it to function improperly. This process, known as *telomere attrition*, plays a crucial role in cellular senescence, tissue damage, and many of the age-related conditions we fear.

～๑

## The Mechanics of Telomere Shortening

Telomeres are made up of repetitive sequences of DNA which don't code for any proteins but act as a buffer zone to protect the essential parts of the chromosome during cell division. Every time a cell divides, the DNA replication machinery must copy the entire genome.

This task falls to an enzyme called DNA polymerase, which acts like a molecular copy machine, building new DNA strands by attaching nucleotides —the building blocks of DNA— to an existing strand. But DNA polymerase has a quirk: it can only add nucleotides to the end of a DNA strand in one specific direction, called the 3' end.

Here's where things get tricky. DNA is made up of two strands running in opposite directions, and during replication, one strand (called the leading strand) is copied smoothly from start to finish. The other strand, known as the lagging strand, is replicated in smaller sections because of the directional limitation of DNA polymerase. When it reaches the very end of this lagging strand, DNA polymerase can't fully replicate the last segment. This leaves a small piece of DNA unfinished after each round of cell division, causing the telomeres to gradually shorten over time — like a candle burning down with each use.

Another factor that accelerates telomere shortening is oxidative stress which results from the accumulation of reactive oxygen species (ROS) in cells — you'll remember these from the chapter on DNA damage. Telomeres are particularly vulnerable to oxidative damage due to their high guanine content, which is one of the four nucleotides in DNA and is especially prone to oxidation.

## Cellular Responses to Telomere Attrition: The Role of DNA Damage Response

Telomeres function like the protective plastic tips on the ends of shoelaces — but what happens when those tips wear down? In cells, the erosion of telomeres doesn't go unnoticed. When telomeres become critically short, they can no longer protect the chromosome ends. The cell perceives this as DNA damage, triggering a DNA damage response (DDR). The activation of this protective mechanism leads to two major cellular outcomes: senescence or apoptosis.

1. **Cellular Senescence**: In most cases, the cell enters a state of senescence — a condition in which the cell permanently stops dividing but remains metabolically active. Senescent cells are sometimes referred to as "zombie cells" because they no longer contribute to tissue regeneration or repair, yet they persist in the body, secreting inflammatory signals that can harm nearby cells. This accumulation of senescent cells in tissues is a significant contributor to the aging process and is linked to age-related diseases such as osteoarthritis, atherosclerosis, and even cancer.

2. **Apoptosis**: In other situations, cells with critically short telomeres may undergo apoptosis, or programmed cell death. This is a self-protective mechanism meant to eliminate cells that could potentially become cancerous due to genomic instability. While apoptosis helps prevent the propagation of damaged cells, excessive apoptosis in tissues can lead to loss of cellular function and contribute to tissue degeneration, another hallmark of aging.

A key player in this response to critically short telomeres is the tumor suppressor protein p53. Often referred to as the "guardian of the genome," p53 is activated when telomeres reach a critical length, triggering cell cycle arrest, senescence, or apoptosis. Without functional p53, cells would continue to divide uncontrollably, leading to the risk of cancerous growth. In fact, mutations in the gene encoding p53 are commonly found in cancer cells, allowing them to evade the protective mechanisms normally triggered by telomere shortening.

~

## Telomerase: The Guardian of Telomeres

While most cells in the human body experience telomere attrition with each division, there is a special enzyme that can reverse this process: telomerase. Telomerase is a ribonucleoprotein that adds repetitive DNA sequences back to the ends of telomeres, effectively rebuilding them and extending the cell's replicative lifespan. This enzyme is made up of two major components:

- **TERT** (telomerase reverse transcriptase), a protein subunit that synthesizes new DNA sequences.
- **TERC** (telomerase RNA component), which provides the template for adding the TTAGGG repeats to the telomeres.

Telomerase is highly active in certain types of cells, including stem cells, germ cells (which give rise to sperm and eggs), and cancer cells. In these cells, telomerase ensures that telomeres remain long enough to support continuous cell division. For example, stem cells must divide frequently to maintain tissue health and regeneration, so telomerase activity allows them to replenish tissues without running into the problem of telomere shortening. In contrast, most somatic cells — the cells that make up the bulk of the body's tissues — have little to no telomerase activity. As a result, telomere attrition in these cells limits their ability to divide, which eventually leads to aging and tissue degeneration.

In cancer cells, telomerase becomes hijacked to fuel uncontrolled cell division. By continuously rebuilding their telomeres, cancer cells effectively become "immortal," allowing them to divide indefinitely and form tumors. This has led to a complex question in aging research: Can telomerase be reactivated in normal cells to extend their lifespan without triggering cancer? While boosting telomerase in humans remains a theoretical possibility, it comes with risks, as its uncontrolled activation could promote the formation of new tumors.

~⁹

## The Shelterin Complex: Protecting Chromosome Ends

One of the most fascinating aspects of telomere biology is the shelterin complex, a group of six proteins that bind to and protect telomeres from being recognized as DNA breaks. These proteins play a vital role in preventing unwanted activation of the DNA damage response and ensuring the proper replication of telomeres.

The shelterin complex includes:

- **TRF1** and **TRF2** (telomeric repeat-binding factors 1 and 2), which bind directly to the telomeric DNA and play essential roles in maintaining telomere structure.

- **POT1** (protection of telomeres 1), which binds to the single-stranded overhang of the telomere and helps control access to telomerase.

- **TIN2, TPP1,** and **Rap1** which help link the components of the shelterin complex together and regulate telomere length and protection.

Without the shelterin complex, the ends of chromosomes would be recognized as double-strand breaks, triggering a damaging DNA repair response. TRF2, in particular, prevents the formation of end-to-end chromosome fusions, which would lead to catastrophic genomic instability. In this way, the shelterin complex ensures that telomeres are properly maintained and protected throughout the cell's life, allowing cells to avoid activating detrimental damage responses prematurely.

## T-Loop Formation: The Final Layer of Protection

In addition to being protected by the shelterin complex, telomeres adopt a unique structure known as the T-loop in which the single-stranded overhang at the very end of the telomere loops back and tucks into the double-stranded portion of the telomeric DNA — you can think of this like tying a knot in your shoelaces to stop them from coming apart. This looped structure further conceals the chromosome ends, preventing them from being mistaken for DNA damage.

The T-loop is stabilized by the shelterin proteins described above, which help telomere ends remain "hidden" from the DNA repair machinery. By forming this protective loop, telomeres are able to guard the chromosome ends during each round of replication, ensuring that cells can divide for as long as their telomeres allow.

~❧

## Telomere Attrition: The Balance of Aging and Disease

Telomere attrition is a fundamental process that balances cellular division and genomic protection. When telomeres are well-maintained by telomerase and shelterin, cells can continue dividing, repairing tissues, and supporting bodily functions. But as telomeres shorten and protective mechanisms weaken, the resulting cellular dysfunction drives aging, tissue degeneration, and the onset of age-related diseases like cardiovascular disease, immune senescence, and neurodegeneration.

The decline of telomere length sets the stage for many of the challenges we face in old age, but understanding the intricate biology of telomeres has opened the door to new strategies for improving health and longevity. While we can't stop the clock on telomere attrition entirely, ongoing research raises the possibility that we may one day be able to slow the process. I will dive into more detail about this in a later part of the book — stay tuned.

# CHAPTER 5

# Epigenetic Alterations: The Fading Instructions of Youth

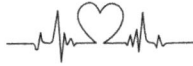

—⎍ᢣ♡₂ᢣ⎍—

Think of your DNA as the hardware of a computer — the physical foundation that holds all the data necessary to run the system. Epigenetics, on the other hand, acts as the software — the programming that tells the hardware what to do. While the hardware remains relatively stable, the software is dynamic, constantly updating and adjusting the system's functions. Epigenetic modifications serve as "on/off switches" for genes, determining which genes are active and which are silenced at any given time. Over time, as we age, this finely tuned software begins to malfunction. The switches flip randomly, turning some genes off that should remain on and vice versa, causing cells to lose their identity and function. This gradual breakdown of epigenetic regulation leads to the deterioration of tissues and the development of age-related diseases, making epigenetic alterations a central hallmark of aging.

Epigenetics refers to modifications that affect gene activity without altering the underlying DNA sequence. Unlike genetic mutations, which directly change the structure of DNA, epigenetic changes are like notes written in the margins, influencing how genes are expressed. Over time, the accumulation of these changes can lead to a loss of cellular function and, ultimately, contribute to the aging process. But how does this happen, and what mechanisms are at play in this age-related breakdown of genetic instructions?

~●

## Understanding Epigenetic Modifications

There are several types of epigenetic modifications, but three major mechanisms are central to the regulation of gene expression: DNA methylation, histone modification, and non-coding RNAs. Each plays a vital role in determining how genes are activated or silenced in different cells. You can think of these mechanisms as the software engineers of the body's genetic system — they decide which parts of the code should be activated and which should remain dormant, ensuring the proper functioning of the cellular machinery.

- **DNA Methylation**: DNA methylation acts as a lock on certain parts of the genetic code. Small molecules, called methyl groups, are added to DNA at specific sites, essentially turning genes off by making them unreadable. In a young and healthy system, these locks are applied only to the genes that should remain silent. But as we age, the programming starts to malfunction, causing some genes that should be active to get locked away, while others that should be silenced get mistakenly activated. This can lead to cellular dysfunction, contributing to age-related conditions such as cancer. Over time, this faulty "locking" mechanism disrupts the balance of gene expression.

  ▪ **Histone Modification**: If DNA methylation is the lock, then histone modification is more like a dimmer switch. DNA doesn't float freely in the nucleus — instead, it's wrapped around proteins called histones, which help package and organize the DNA. When chemical groups are added to histones, they can tighten or loosen their grip on the DNA. A tight grip means that the genes are hidden, like files stored deep in a computer system, making them inaccessible. A looser grip makes the DNA more accessible, allowing genes to be turned on. In youth, histone modifications keep this system running smoothly, ensuring that the right files (genes) are open and the wrong ones are closed. But as with DNA methylation, aging causes the system to go haywire, leaving some important genes closed when they should be open, and vice versa.

- **Non-Coding RNAs**: Not all RNA is used to translate DNA into proteins. A large portion of the human genome produces *non-coding RNAs (ncRNAs)*, which act as the regulatory tools that help manage the genetic system. These molecules are like little software patches that manage how the cell uses its resources. Some non-coding RNAs, like microRNAs, can bind to messenger RNA (the molecule that carries genetic instructions to make proteins), effectively preventing certain proteins from being produced. Over time, the expression of these regulatory RNAs becomes erratic, leading to further problems in gene regulation. It's as if these patches start malfunctioning, causing the genetic system to produce too much or too little of key proteins.

## The Erosion of Epigenetic Fidelity with Age

Just as a finely tuned instrument can fall out of harmony over time, so too can the epigenetic mechanisms that regulate gene expression.

In youth, our cells maintain what is called "epigenetic fidelity" — the ability to preserve precise patterns of gene expression. This fidelity is crucial for keeping cells in their proper functional state. For instance, a liver cell knows it is a liver cell because its genes are marked to express liver-specific proteins, while other genes that would make it behave like a skin or brain cell are silenced.

However, as we age, this epigenetic fidelity starts to degrade. DNA methylation patterns become less stable, histone modifications grow erratic, and non-coding RNA expression becomes dysregulated. This gradual breakdown leads to the loss of cellular identity. A once-healthy liver cell may begin expressing genes more characteristic of other tissues, such as muscle or skin. This cellular confusion contributes to tissue dysfunction and the decline of organ systems.

One of the most notable examples of this epigenetic drift is seen in cancer cells. As normal cells accumulate epigenetic alterations with age, they are more likely to undergo malignant transformations. Many cancers are characterized by widespread changes in DNA methylation, where tumor-suppressing genes are silenced, and oncogenes (cancer-promoting genes) are activated. Thus, the gradual erosion of the epigenetic landscape is a critical driver not only of aging but also of age-related diseases like cancer.

~~

## Key Players in Epigenetic Aging

Much like any complex software system, the body's epigenetic regulation is managed by a variety of key tools and components. These "key players" are the enzymes and proteins that write, erase, and read the epigenetic marks that determine gene activity:

- **DNA Methyltransferases (DNMTs):** Think of DNA methyltransferases as the programmers that add locks to specific parts of the DNA. These enzymes are responsible for placing methyl groups onto the DNA, effectively switching off certain genes. In younger cells, DNA methyltransferases help ensure that methylation patterns are precise and stable. However, as we age, these enzymes can misplace their marks, leading to faulty gene silencing. This is like a software program where some of the commands are executed incorrectly, causing the system to malfunction. In aged cells, this malfunction can lead to the inappropriate activation of genes that promote cancer or the silencing of genes critical for normal cell function.

- **Histone-Modifying Enzymes:** Just as DNA methyltransferases control the locks, histone-modifying enzymes manage the dimmer switches of gene expression. Two important types of enzymes are histone acetyltransferases (HATs) and histone deacetylases (HDACs). HATs add acetyl groups to histones, loosening their hold on the DNA and making genes more accessible for transcription. On the other hand, HDACs remove acetyl groups, tightening the grip and silencing gene expression. When these enzymes are working well, they ensure that the right genes are accessible at the right time. But with age, the balance between the two becomes disrupted, causing improper regulation of gene activity.

- **Sirtuins:** Sirtuins are the "maintenance crew" of the epigenetic system, known for their role in DNA repair and maintaining genomic stability. These proteins are often referred to as longevity genes because of their ability to slow down some aspects of aging. Sirtuins primarily work by removing acetyl groups from histones (like HDACs), keeping the chromatin structure in good shape. But beyond that, sirtuins help protect the genome from damage caused by environmental stressors and oxidative stress. As we age, sirtuin levels decrease, which means less protection and more errors in the system. It's as though the maintenance crew has become understaffed, leaving many of the critical repairs undone.

- **Polycomb and Trithorax Complexes**: The Polycomb group proteins are responsible for gene silencing — they keep certain regions of the DNA tightly packed and inaccessible. In contrast, the Trithorax group proteins promote gene expression, keeping chromatin open and allowing genes to be turned on. In youth, these two systems work in balance, ensuring that genes are expressed or silenced as needed. But with age, this balance is disrupted, leading to inappropriate activation or repression of genes.

~❧

## The Role of Epigenetic Alterations in Disease

Epigenetic alterations don't just contribute to the general aging process — they are also implicated in many age-related diseases. As the epigenome becomes increasingly disorganized, the risk of developing chronic diseases rises. For example, changes in DNA methylation have been linked to Alzheimer's disease, where key genes involved in memory and cognition become improperly silenced or activated. Similarly, epigenetic dysregulation plays a role in cardiovascular disease, where the expression of genes that control inflammation and blood vessel function becomes altered with age.

Additionally, the loss of epigenetic regulation contributes to *immune senescence*, a decline in immune function that makes older adults more susceptible to infections and less responsive to vaccines. As epigenetic drift progresses, immune cells lose their ability to mount effective responses to pathogens, leading to a higher risk of disease and slower recovery times.

~~●

## The Promise of Epigenetic Research

So, after all that, why should you care about epigenetic alterations? Well, they are one of the most fascinating hallmarks of aging because they offer both a window into how we age and a potential avenue for intervention. Unlike genetic mutations, which are difficult to reverse, epigenetic changes are potentially malleable. Emerging therapies, such as drugs that target DNA methylation or histone modifications, offer the exciting possibility of restoring youthful gene expression patterns in aging cells.

While the field is still in its early stages, the idea of "reprogramming" our cells to reverse epigenetic drift could one day transform how we approach aging and age-related diseases. The key lies in understanding the complexity of these mechanisms and learning how to manipulate them safely.

# CHAPTER 6

# Loss of Proteostasis: The Breakdown of Cellular Maintenance

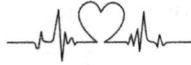

Imagine your body as a factory that never stops running, day and night, tirelessly producing and maintaining the proteins that make life possible. Proteins are the essential machinery that keeps everything functioning. They're responsible for nearly every task inside your cells, from regulating your metabolism to repairing damaged DNA. But, just like any complex factory, things can go wrong. Over time, as wear and tear accumulate, the quality control mechanisms of this factory start to fail. This breakdown in maintenance and repair is known as loss of proteostasis — a hallmark of aging that leads to cellular dysfunction, tissue damage, and, eventually, disease.

Proteostasis, or protein homeostasis, is the system responsible for making sure proteins are properly produced, folded, and discarded when they're no longer useful. In a young, healthy body, this system runs smoothly, with faulty or damaged proteins quickly identified and either repaired or removed. But as we age, this process falters. The result? Misfolded proteins accumulate, and the cellular machinery begins to malfunction. It's a slow but relentless decline, like a well-oiled machine gradually breaking down, until it can no longer perform the tasks it once could.

## The Role of Proteins and Protein Folding

Proteins are the workhorses of the cell, but they don't start out in their final, functional form. Instead, they begin as long chains of amino acids that must fold into specific three-dimensional shapes to do their job — this folding process is critical, as the structure of a protein determines its function. Like a misassembled tool, if a protein isn't folded correctly, it can't function. Worse, misfolded proteins can become toxic to the cell, sticking together to form clumps or aggregates that interfere with normal cellular processes.

In healthy cells, the process of protein folding is carefully monitored by *molecular chaperones,* specialized proteins that assist in the correct folding of newly synthesized proteins. These chaperones act like quality control inspectors, ensuring that each protein is folded correctly before it is allowed to enter the cell's "workforce." If a protein cannot be properly folded, the cell will typically send it for degradation through a process known as *proteolysis.* This ensures that faulty proteins don't accumulate and cause harm.

As we age, the ability to maintain this system diminishes. The production of molecular chaperones decreases, and the mechanisms for degrading damaged proteins become less efficient. Misfolded proteins begin to accumulate, forming aggregates that can interfere with normal cellular functions. These protein aggregates are a hallmark of several age-related diseases, including Alzheimer's, Parkinson's, and Huntington's disease, where clumps of misfolded proteins are associated with widespread neuronal damage.

## Cellular Mechanisms of Proteostasis

There are two major systems within the cell responsible for maintaining proteostasis: the *ubiquitin-proteasome system (UPS)* and *autophagy*. Both systems play critical roles in ensuring that damaged, misfolded, or excess proteins are removed from the cell, maintaining a clean and functional internal environment.

- **Ubiquitin-Proteasome System (UPS)**: The UPS is the primary system for degrading short-lived and damaged proteins. Proteins that are marked for degradation are tagged with a molecule called ubiquitin, which acts like a molecular "garbage tag" signaling that the protein should be disposed of. Once tagged, these proteins are sent to the *proteasome*, a massive protein complex that acts like a molecular shredder, breaking the protein down into its component parts so they can be recycled.

- **Autophagy**: The second line of defense is autophagy, which means "self-eating." This is the cell's way of clearing out larger protein aggregates or damaged organelles that the proteasome cannot handle. In autophagy, unwanted cellular material is engulfed by a membrane, forming a structure known as an *autophagosome*. This autophagosome then fuses with a *lysosome*, an organelle filled with enzymes that break down and digest the contents. Autophagy is essential for maintaining cellular health, particularly during periods of stress or nutrient scarcity, when the cell may need to recycle components to survive.

When these systems falter, the cell is left with an overload of damaged and misfolded proteins. This buildup not only disrupts cellular function but also triggers inflammatory responses and oxidative stress, further accelerating the aging process.

~⊱

## The Impact of Protein Aggregates on Aging

The accumulation of misfolded and aggregated proteins is not just a byproduct of aging; it is a driving force behind many age-related diseases. These protein aggregates can disrupt cellular functions in several ways. First, they can interfere with normal cellular processes by physically blocking pathways or organelles. For example, in neurodegenerative diseases, protein aggregates often disrupt the transport of molecules along the axons of neurons, impairing communication between nerve cells.

Second, these aggregates can induce inflammation. When cells recognize the presence of misfolded proteins, they often trigger an immune response, releasing inflammatory signals in an attempt to clear the harmful material. While this response is meant to protect the cell, chronic inflammation caused by persistent protein aggregates can lead to tissue damage and contribute to the progression of diseases like atherosclerosis and arthritis.

Lastly, the accumulation of damaged proteins increases oxidative stress within cells. As proteins become oxidized, they lose their functionality and become more prone to misfolding. This creates a vicious cycle where oxidative stress leads to more misfolded proteins, which in turn generate more oxidative stress, accelerating the aging process.

~⊱

## Why Does Proteostasis Fail with Age?

If proteostasis is so essential for maintaining cellular health, why does it fail as we get older? There are several reasons, and they all point to the same conclusion: aging cells simply can't keep up with the demands of protein maintenance.

First, the production of molecular chaperones declines with age, reducing the cell's ability to properly fold proteins. Without enough chaperones to keep the process running smoothly, misfolded proteins start to accumulate.

At the same time, the activity of the proteasome — the cell's main garbage disposal system — also declines. Studies have shown that proteasome function decreases significantly in older cells, meaning damaged proteins that should be destroyed end up sticking around, gumming up the works.

To make matters worse, autophagy becomes less efficient with age. This is particularly problematic because autophagy is the only way cells can clear out large aggregates of misfolded proteins. When autophagy slows down, these toxic protein clumps start to accumulate, leading to the kind of cellular dysfunction we see in diseases like Alzheimer's, where amyloid-beta plaques form in the brain, or Parkinson's, where alpha-synuclein clumps together to form Lewy bodies.

Oxidative stress, another hallmark of aging, also plays a role in the loss of proteostasis. Reactive oxygen species (ROS), which are produced as byproducts of normal cellular metabolism, can damage proteins, making them more prone to misfolding. As we age, the balance between ROS production and the cell's ability to neutralize these harmful molecules tips in favor of oxidative damage. This creates a vicious cycle: damaged proteins generate more oxidative stress, which in turn leads to more misfolding and aggregation.

~~●

## The Role of Proteostasis in Age-Related Diseases

The loss of proteostasis is a critical factor in the development of many age-related diseases. Neurodegenerative disorders like Alzheimer's, Parkinson's, and Huntington's disease are perhaps the most well-known examples of conditions where proteostasis failure plays a central role. In these diseases, the accumulation of misfolded proteins, such as amyloid-beta, tau, and alpha-synuclein, leads to widespread neuronal damage and loss of brain function.

But proteostasis failure is not limited to the nervous system. In the cardiovascular system, the buildup of damaged proteins contributes to the development of *atherosclerosis*, where protein aggregates accumulate in the walls of arteries, leading to inflammation and plaque formation. Similarly, in skeletal muscle, the loss of proteostasis has been linked to *sarcopenia*, the age-related loss of muscle mass and strength. As misfolded proteins accumulate in muscle cells, they impair cellular function and reduce the ability of muscles to regenerate, leading to weakness and frailty.

# CHAPTER 7

# Disabled Macroautophagy: When Cellular Cleanup Breaks Down

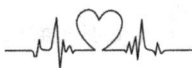

—ᴧᴧᏉᎬᴧᴧ—

In the previous chapter, I introduced the concept of (macro)autophagy as part of the broader system of proteostasis — the cellular mechanisms that maintain protein quality and remove damaged components. Since autophagy plays such an integral role in this cleanup process, it's impossible to talk about proteostasis without mentioning it. To avoid redundancy, I'll focus on the more specific aspects of autophagy failure and its direct connection to aging in this chapter.

While autophagy's role in maintaining cellular health was previously recognized, it was only in a recent update to the hallmarks of aging that disabled macroautophagy was identified as a distinct contributor to aging. So, what exactly goes wrong when macroautophagy becomes impaired, and why does this failure play such a critical role in aging?

～๑

## The Breakdown of Macroautophagy in Aging

A quick recap: autophagy is not about destruction, but renewal. Imagine it as the ultimate recycling program. When cells encounter damaged proteins, organelles, or other cellular waste, autophagy steps in to break down these components and repurpose them for new construction. It's a system designed to keep the cell running efficiently, much like a factory repurposing scrap materials to avoid waste and ensure smooth production.

Surprise surprise, as we age this recycling system begins to malfunction. The machinery that once maintained cellular cleanliness begins to sputter. Autophagosomes form less frequently, and even when they do, the process of delivering their cargo to lysosomes becomes sluggish. The lysosomes themselves may also become less effective, no longer able to break down the material they're given. As a result, damaged proteins, misfolded molecules, and malfunctioning organelles accumulate inside the cell, contributing to a cascade of cellular dysfunction.

But why does macroautophagy break down with age? One key issue is the gradual reduction in the expression of *autophagy-related genes*, known as "ATG genes." These genes encode proteins that are critical for various steps in the autophagic process, from the formation of autophagosomes to the fusion of autophagosomes with lysosomes. As the expression of these genes wanes, so too does the cell's ability to carry out autophagy effectively.

Additionally, changes in the nutrient-sensing pathways that regulate autophagy also play a role in its decline. The *mTOR (mechanistic target of rapamycin) pathway*, for example, is a central regulator of cell growth and metabolism, and it is highly responsive to nutrient availability. In times of nutrient abundance, mTOR activity is high, and autophagy is suppressed. In contrast, during periods of nutrient scarcity, mTOR activity decreases, allowing autophagy to ramp up. mTOR signaling becomes increasingly dysregulated in old age, often remaining elevated even when it should be downregulated to allow for autophagy. This persistent activation of mTOR interrupts the autophagic process, preventing cells from clearing out damaged components.

~∂

## The Accumulation of Cellular Waste: A Growing Problem

When autophagy fails, the consequences are far-reaching. Without the ability to properly degrade and recycle damaged cellular components, cells become overwhelmed by waste. Misfolded proteins, damaged mitochondria, and other cellular debris accumulate, creating a toxic environment that impairs cell function. This buildup of waste leads to *cellular senescence*, a state in which cells stop dividing and enter a sort of limbo. While senescent cells don't die, they secrete harmful inflammatory signals that damage surrounding cells, contributing to tissue dysfunction and chronic inflammation — a hallmark of aging known as "inflammaging."

The failure to remove damaged mitochondria, in particular, is a significant contributor to the aging process. Mitochondria are the engines that power the cell, generating energy in the form of ATP. But as they age, mitochondria become less efficient and more prone to damage, producing harmful *reactive oxygen species* that can wreak havoc on cellular structures. Normally, damaged mitochondria are removed through a specialized form of autophagy called *mitophagy*, which targets and degrades faulty mitochondria. However, with the decline in autophagic efficiency, these defective mitochondria accumulate, amplifying oxidative stress and accelerating cellular aging.

The ripple effects of disabled macroautophagy extend beyond individual cells. At the tissue and organ level, the inability to clear damaged components leads to the gradual decline of organ function. For example, in the liver, which plays a central role in detoxifying the body, impaired autophagy can lead to the buildup of damaged proteins and fats, contributing to conditions like non-alcoholic fatty liver disease (NAFLD). In the immune system, the failure of autophagy to clear out dysfunctional immune cells weakens the body's ability to fight off infections, making older adults more susceptible to diseases.

## A New Hallmark of Aging: Why Macroautophagy Matters

The recognition of disabled macroautophagy as a hallmark of aging is relatively recent, but its importance is clear. As researchers have delved deeper into the mechanisms of aging, the role of autophagy in maintaining cellular health has become increasingly apparent. The addition of this hallmark highlights a critical aspect of aging that was previously underappreciated: the failure of cells to clean up after themselves.

Understanding how to preserve and restore autophagy could unlock new ways to extend both lifespan and healthspan, offering hope for a future where the burden of age-related diseases is significantly reduced.

One reason why macroautophagy is gaining more attention is its potential as a therapeutic target. Unlike some other hallmarks of aging, which involve irreversible damage (such as genomic instability), macroautophagy is a process that can potentially be restored. Experimental studies have shown that boosting autophagy can extend lifespan in various model organisms, from yeast to mice. In particular, interventions that suppress mTOR activity, such as caloric restriction or drugs like **rapamycin,** have been shown to enhance autophagic function, reducing the accumulation of damaged proteins and organelles.

# CHAPTER 8

# Deregulated Nutrient-Sensing: When the Cellular Fuel Gauge Fails

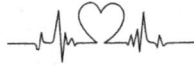

—∿𝓵∿♡²∿𝓵∿—

Cells are like finely tuned machines, adjusting their output based on the availability of fuel — glucose, amino acids, fatty acids — and adapting to fluctuations in supply and demand. This delicate balance is regulated by a series of nutrient-sensing pathways that act like cellular fuel gauges, ensuring that the body functions efficiently, storing energy when food is abundant and conserving resources when it's scarce.

When we're young, these nutrient-sensing pathways respond appropriately to changes in energy and nutrient availability, keeping the body's metabolism in check. But as we age, this regulation begins to falter. These once finely tuned sensors become less responsive, leading to deregulated nutrient-sensing. When nutrient-sensing goes awry, it disrupts the balance between growth and repair, accelerating aging and contributing to age-related diseases like diabetes, cardiovascular disease, and cancer.

～❧

## The Four Key Pathways

At the core of nutrient-sensing are four main pathways: *insulin and insulin-like growth factor 1 (IGF-1), mTOR, AMP-activated protein kinase (AMPK),* and *sirtuins.* These pathways regulate how cells respond to nutrients, energy, and stress, determining whether cells should build and grow or slow down and repair.

Imagine a factory that alternates between full production mode when resources are abundant and repair mode when the machinery needs maintenance. Nutrient-sensing pathways are the managers that make these calls. But when these systems become deregulated, as they do with aging, the factory keeps running on overdrive, burning through resources and allowing the machinery to wear down. The result is accelerated cellular damage, inflammation, and metabolic disorders.

~⌘

## Insulin and IGF-1: The Growth Pathway

One of the most important nutrient-sensing systems in the body is the insulin/IGF-1 pathway. Insulin, secreted by the pancreas in response to high blood sugar, helps cells absorb glucose and convert it into energy or store it for later use. IGF-1, closely related to insulin, is a hormone that promotes cell growth and survival, particularly in muscle and bone tissues. Together, insulin and IGF-1 act as growth signals, telling cells that it's time to use nutrients for energy and growth.

However, with age, cells become less sensitive to insulin, a condition known as insulin resistance. As a result, the body needs to produce more and more insulin to maintain stable blood sugar levels. Over time, this chronic overproduction of insulin leads to the dysfunction of nutrient-sensing pathways, driving conditions like type 2 diabetes and obesity. In a vicious cycle, insulin resistance contributes to inflammation and oxidative stress, which further impair nutrient sensing and accelerate the aging process.

In addition to insulin resistance, the IGF-1 pathway also becomes dysregulated with age. IGF-1 is crucial for promoting cell growth, but when this pathway is overactivated, it encourages the continuous proliferation of cells — a process linked to cancer and age-related tissue degeneration. In animal studies, reducing IGF-1 signaling has been shown to extend lifespan, suggesting that fine-tuning this pathway may be key to promoting longevity.

~~

## mTOR: The Growth Command Center

While insulin and IGF-1 are responsible for responding to nutrient availability, mTOR (mechanistic target of rapamycin) acts as the central growth command center, regulating how cells use these nutrients. mTOR is highly responsive to amino acids, and it plays a critical role in promoting cell growth, protein synthesis, and metabolism. When nutrients are abundant, mTOR signals to cells that it's time to grow and proliferate.

But mTOR's growth-promoting effects come at a cost. Just as a car engine that runs too fast for too long eventually breaks down, mTOR's constant activation leads to cellular wear and tear. This overdrive mode, especially in the context of excessive nutrient intake, accelerates aging by preventing cells from switching into repair and maintenance modes. Persistent mTOR activity inhibits autophagy — the cellular "recycling" process that clears out damaged proteins and organelles — leading to the buildup of cellular waste and dysfunction.

Interestingly, mTOR inhibition has been linked to lifespan extension in various organisms, from yeast to mammals. Rapamycin, a drug that inhibits mTOR, has shown promise in extending lifespan and improving healthspan by shifting the balance away from constant growth toward repair. In essence, reducing mTOR activity allows the cell to slow down, repair damage, and conserve energy — a strategy that seems to promote longevity in the long run.

~❦

## AMPK: The Cellular Energy Sensor

Where insulin, IGF-1, and mTOR promote growth in response to nutrient abundance, AMPK (AMP-activated protein kinase) acts as the counterbalance. AMPK is like the cell's fuel gauge, detecting when energy levels are low and activating pathways that conserve energy and promote repair. When cells are low on energy — for example, during exercise or fasting — AMPK is activated, signaling the cell to switch from growth to maintenance.

AMPK helps cells survive by enhancing mitochondrial function, promoting fatty acid oxidation, and stimulating autophagy. By activating these pathways, AMPK ensures that cells can efficiently manage their energy resources and eliminate damaged components. Yet with age, AMPK activity declines, reducing the cell's ability to respond to energy stress. This decline in AMPK activity is linked to metabolic diseases like obesity and type 2 diabetes, as well as a reduction in the overall ability of cells to repair and maintain themselves.

Studies have shown that boosting AMPK activity can improve metabolic health and extend lifespan in animal models.

Interventions like caloric restriction, exercise, and certain compounds (such as *metformin*, a diabetes drug) activate AMPK, mimicking the effects of nutrient scarcity and promoting the health benefits associated with a more balanced nutrient-sensing system. I'll dive into these strategies in more detail later in the book.

~~✎~~

## Sirtuins: The Longevity Regulators

*Sirtuins*, often referred to as the "longevity genes," are a family of proteins that regulate cellular stress responses, DNA repair, and metabolism. Like AMPK, sirtuins are activated by nutrient scarcity, particularly during *fasting* or *caloric restriction*. These proteins play a key role in promoting cellular resilience, helping cells survive and repair themselves under stress. Sirtuins regulate mitochondrial function, enhance DNA repair, and stimulate autophagy, making them essential for maintaining cellular health as we age.

One of the most well-known sirtuins, *SIRT1*, is involved in regulating metabolic processes and protecting us from oxidative stress. It has been shown that activating SIRT1 can extend lifespan in various organisms by enhancing the cell's ability to cope with damage and conserve energy. Sirtuins are also influenced by the availability of NAD+ (nicotinamide adenine dinucleotide), a molecule that declines with age and is essential for sirtuin activity. As NAD+ levels drop, sirtuin activity decreases, contributing to cellular aging and the decline in metabolic health.

Efforts to boost sirtuin activity through NAD+ precursors, such as nicotinamide riboside (NR) and nicotinamide mononucleotide (NMN), have gained attention in recent years for their potential to slow aging and improve healthspan. These interventions aim to restore the balance of nutrient-sensing pathways, helping cells shift between growth and repair as needed, even in the face of aging.

~●

## The Consequences of Deregulated Nutrient-Sensing

When nutrient-sensing pathways are deregulated, the consequences extend far beyond metabolic disorders. The improper balance between growth and repair accelerates the onset of numerous age-related diseases, including cancer, cardiovascular disease, and neurodegenerative conditions. Chronic overactivation of growth pathways like mTOR and IGF-1 promotes the uncontrolled proliferation of cells, increasing the risk of cancer. Meanwhile, the suppression of repair mechanisms like autophagy leads to the accumulation of cellular damage, contributing to neurodegeneration and cognitive decline.

Deregulated nutrient-sensing is also closely linked to the development of metabolic syndrome, a cluster of conditions that includes obesity, insulin resistance, high blood pressure, and abnormal cholesterol levels. Metabolic syndrome increases the risk of heart disease, stroke, and diabetes, all of which are more common as we age.

# CHAPTER 9

# Mitochondrial Dysfunction: The Failing Power Plants of Aging Cells

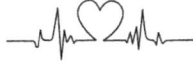

—ᴧᴧᴧ♡ᴧᴧ—

Imagine your cells as tiny cities, bustling with activity, each powered by its own energy grid. The mitochondria are the power plants of this cellular metropolis, supplying the energy needed to keep everything running smoothly. But what happens when those power plants start to break down? When the energy they provide isn't quite enough? This is the story of mitochondrial dysfunction, a key factor in the decline we experience as we grow older.

Mitochondria aren't just the cell's powerhouses; they do far more than churn out energy. They also help regulate metabolism, manage calcium levels, and even decide when a cell should die. But like anything that works day in, day out, mitochondria accumulate damage over time. And as they falter, the effects ripple outward, affecting everything from muscle strength to brain function. In short, as your mitochondria age, so do you.

∿

## How Mitochondria Power the Cell

At the heart of every mitochondrion is the production of *ATP*, or *adenosine triphosphate* — the molecule that fuels almost every cellular activity. Mitochondria generate ATP through *oxidative phosphorylation*, a process that requires a constant flow of electrons across a series of proteins embedded in their inner membrane. This electron transfer system acts like a miniature factory, turning nutrients into usable energy. But, as with any industrial process, there are by-products: in this case, reactive oxygen species (ROS), or free radicals. These molecules are highly reactive and, in small amounts, actually help signal cells to repair themselves. But when too many are produced, they become destructive, damaging proteins, lipids, and even DNA.

In young, healthy cells, mitochondria are equipped to manage this balance. They produce energy efficiently and keep free-radical levels in check. But as we age, mitochondria lose their edge. They become less effective at generating energy, and the production of free radicals skyrockets. This kicks off a downward spiral of damage where mitochondria produce more free radicals, which further damages the mitochondria, in turn leading to even more free radicals.

~❧

## The Snowball Effect of Mitochondrial Damage

One of the reasons mitochondria are so vulnerable is their unique genetic makeup. Mitochondria have their own DNA, separate from the DNA in the cell's nucleus. This *mitochondrial DNA (mtDNA)* is passed down maternally and, crucially, it lacks many of the repair mechanisms that protect nuclear DNA. Over time, as mitochondria churn out energy, their mitochondrial DNA is exposed to high levels of free radicals, which leads to mutations. These mutations further impair mitochondrial function, creating a downward spiral where mitochondria become less and less capable of producing energy efficiently.

Over time, the whole system becomes unreliable: as more mitochondria accumulate damage, they become a drag on the cell, unable to meet the energy demands of tissues, especially those with high energy needs like muscles, the brain, and the heart.

Evidence for the role of mitochondrial DNA mutations in aging comes from studies in model organisms. In mtDNA mutator mice, which carry mutations in the mitochondrial DNA polymerase responsible for copying mitochondrial DNA, there are obvious signs of accelerated aging, with the mice developing symptoms like muscle wasting, hair loss, and reduced fertility at a much earlier age.

## Can We Make New Mitochondria?

The good news is that cells aren't powerless against mitochondrial dysfunction. They have a system in place to create new mitochondria, a process called *mitochondrial biogenesis.* This is where the protein *PGC-1α* comes into play. PGC-1α is like the foreman of the mitochondrial repair shop, coordinating the production of new mitochondria and ensuring they're in working order. But as we age, the efficiency of mitochondrial biogenesis declines. Even though the cell tries to produce fresh, functional mitochondria, the output is lower, and damaged mitochondria still pile up.

So, while our cells do their best to keep up with the wear and tear, aging shifts the balance. This results in a steady decline in the overall energy-producing capacity of our cells, leaving us more prone to fatigue, muscle weakness, and cognitive decline as the tissues most reliant on high energy output begin to falter.

~~9

## The Role of Mitochondrial Dynamics: Fusion and Fission

Mitochondria are not static structures; they're highly dynamic, constantly undergoing cycles of fusion and fission. These processes allow mitochondria to adapt to changing energy demands and repair themselves. Fusion enables mitochondria to share their contents and mix their genetic material, which helps maintain mitochondrial function — essentially, two mitochondria that are damaged or deficient in different ways come together to form one functioning mitochondrion. Fission, on the other hand, allows the cell to isolate damaged sections of mitochondria, which can then be targeted for destruction through a process called *mitophagy*. This constant remodeling helps maintain a healthy population of mitochondria within cells.

But yet again, aging, ever the harbinger of bad news, disrupts this delicate balance between fusion and fission. In aged cells, there is often an increase in fission, leading to a fragmented mitochondrial network that is less efficient at producing energy. At the same time, fusion becomes less effective, reducing the cell's ability to repair damaged mitochondria. The result is a population of small, dysfunctional mitochondria that only add to the cell's energy woes.

~~9

## Mitophagy: Taking Out the Cellular Trash

When a mitochondrion is beyond repair, the cell relies on mitophagy to clean up the mess. Mitophagy is a specialized form of autophagy that specifically targets damaged mitochondria for degradation. It's like the cell's garbage disposal system: when a mitochondrion can no longer function, it's marked for destruction and broken down into its component parts, which are then recycled.

The *PINK1/Parkin* pathway is one of the main regulators of mitophagy. When a mitochondrion is damaged, the PINK1 protein accumulates on its outer membrane, signaling for Parkin to tag the mitochondrion for disposal. This pathway works well in young, healthy cells, but just like the other systems we've discussed, it becomes less efficient with age. Damaged mitochondria accumulate faster than they can be cleared, leading to a buildup of dysfunctional mitochondria, increased oxidative stress, and further cellular damage.

~~&

## Mitochondrial Dysfunction and Age-Related Disease

The breakdown of mitochondrial function doesn't just cause fatigue or muscle weakness; it's a major driver of age-related diseases. For example, in Alzheimer's disease, mitochondrial dysfunction contributes to the buildup of amyloid-beta plaques and tau tangles in the brain, accelerating cognitive decline. In Parkinson's disease, damaged mitochondria in neurons lead to the loss of dopamine-producing cells, which are critical for movement control. And in the heart, where energy demands are constantly high, mitochondrial dysfunction is linked to heart failure and other cardiovascular diseases.

The accumulation of damaged mitochondria also ramps up inflammation, as dysfunctional mitochondria release signals that trigger the immune system. This leads to inflammaging, the chronic, low-grade inflammation that characterizes aging and plays a role in many age-related conditions. It's as though the body's internal alarms are constantly going off, creating a state of stress that speeds up the aging process.

# CHAPTER 10

# Cellular Senescence: The Cell's Final Countdown

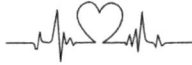

—₁ᴸᴸ♡₂ᴸᴸ—

Picture a bustling city where workers busily carry out their tasks, keeping everything running smoothly. Now imagine some of those workers suddenly stop working—not because they've been fired or retired, but because they've simply paused mid-task and refuse to leave. Over time, they begin to pile up, causing congestion and disrupting the city's flow. This is an analogy for *cellular senescence*, a biological process where cells stop dividing but don't die, lingering within the tissues. Initially a protective mechanism, senescence halts the growth of damaged or stressed cells, preventing them from becoming cancerous. But, like a double-edged sword, these cells can also become toxic to their environment, contributing to aging and a host of age-related diseases.

First discovered in the early 1960s by Leonard Hayflick, senescence was initially understood as a limit to cell division, aptly called the *Hayflick limit*. When cells reach the end of their division capacity, usually due to shortened telomeres (the protective ends of chromosomes), they enter a permanent growth arrest known as replicative senescence. But as research unfolded, scientists found that telomere shortening isn't the only trigger for senescence. Cells can also enter this state due to other stressors, such as DNA damage, oxidative stress, or oncogene activation.

~~●

## The Biology Behind Cellular Senescence

At its core, cellular senescence is a stress response. When cells accumulate too much damage, they activate tumor-suppressor pathways like *p53* and *p16INK4a*, which halt cell division. This is the cell's way of preventing the propagation of damaged or cancer-prone cells. However, while the cell may stop dividing, it remains metabolically active, and this is where things get complicated.

Once a cell enters senescence, it undergoes a host of changes, including alterations in gene expression and protein production. One of the most harmful outcomes is the secretion of pro-inflammatory molecules, growth factors, and enzymes — a toxic mix collectively known as the *senescence-associated secretory phenotype* or SASP. Importantly, the effects of SASP can spread beyond the senescent cell itself, inducing inflammation in neighboring cells and even promoting senescence in nearby healthy cells. A bit like that one rotten fruit that causes the rest of the fruit basket to spoil as well.

~~●

## The Role of Senescence in Aging

While cellular senescence plays an important role in preventing cancer in younger organisms, the story changes as we age. As more cells become senescent, they accumulate in tissues and organs, releasing SASP factors that lead to chronic inflammation, tissue degradation, and dysfunction. This accumulation of senescent cells is one of the key drivers of "inflammaging," a chronic, low-grade inflammation that is characteristic of old-age.

Over time, senescent cells contribute to the weakening of tissues and organs. In the skin, senescent fibroblasts decrease the production of collagen, leading to wrinkles and thinning skin. In joints, senescent cells promote inflammation, contributing to conditions like osteoarthritis. In blood vessels, they contribute to atherosclerosis, the stiffening of arteries, increasing the risk of cardiovascular disease.

## The Double-Edged Sword: Benefits of Senescence?

Senescence isn't all bad. In fact, as mentioned, it's a vital defense mechanism against cancer. By halting the division of damaged cells, senescence prevents the runaway cell growth that leads to tumors. It also plays a role in wound healing, where senescent cells help to initiate tissue repair by secreting factors that attract immune cells to the site of injury.

Moreover, during embryonic development, senescence is essential for proper tissue patterning. In this context, it's a finely tuned process, controlled and temporary, ensuring that organs and tissues develop correctly.

However, the downside emerges later in life when the accumulation of senescent cells begins to outweigh their benefits. As the immune system ages, it becomes less effective at clearing these cells, allowing them to linger and wreak havoc.

## Mechanisms Driving Cellular Senescence

At the molecular level, senescence is triggered by various forms of cellular stress. The most well-known is telomere shortening, which occurs naturally as cells divide. Every time a cell replicates, its telomeres get shorter until they reach a critical length, at which point the cell stops dividing. This process is like a countdown timer built into our cells, limiting how many times they can replicate before entering senescence.

But telomere shortening isn't the only trigger. DNA damage—from environmental factors like UV radiation or internal sources like oxidative stress—can also push a cell into senescence. In fact, the accumulation of DNA damage over time is one of the primary drivers of aging. When DNA is damaged, it activates a cascade of signals called the *DNA damage response (DDR)*, which works to halt the cell cycle and initiate repair. If the damage is too severe to fix, the cell enters senescence.

Another pathway leading to senescence is *oncogene activation.* Oncogenes are mutated versions of normal genes that promote cancer. When cells experience abnormal growth signals from these oncogenes, they can enter a state of *oncogene-induced senescence (OIS)*, effectively stopping cancer in its tracks. That said, the same mechanisms that stop cancer growth also contribute to the aging process when they become dysregulated.

~~

## Cellular Senescence and Disease

Senescence is closely linked to many age-related diseases. One of the most well-studied connections is between senescence and cardiovascular disease. Senescent cells in blood vessels promote the formation of plaques that lead to atherosclerosis, a major risk factor for heart attacks and strokes. These cells also contribute to the stiffening of blood vessels, making it harder for the heart to pump blood efficiently.

In the context of cancer, the relationship is complex. While senescence prevents the growth of cancer cells, the SASP produced by senescent cells can also create a pro-inflammatory environment that supports tumor growth. Additionally, the persistence of senescent cells in the tumor microenvironment can hinder the body's ability to clear cancerous cells, making some tumors more resistant to treatment.

In the brain, senescent cells are implicated in neurodegenerative diseases like Alzheimer's and Parkinson's. Senescent immune cells in the brain release inflammatory molecules that damage neurons, accelerating cognitive decline. Senescence in brain-support cells, such as astrocytes and microglia, also contributes to this process, creating a toxic environment that worsens neurodegeneration.

~~✣~~

## Senescence — A Force for Good and Evil

Cellular senescence is a paradox of aging. It is both a protector and a destroyer, halting the growth of damaged cells but also contributing to the wear and tear that leads to aging. The future of longevity may well lie in our ability to manage this delicate balance, keeping the protective aspects of senescence while minimizing its harmful effects.

# CHAPTER 11

# Stem Cell Exhaustion: When the Body's Reserves Run Dry

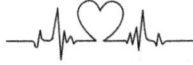

—ιψ♡2ψι—

Your body is like a ship, sailing through the seas of life. At the beginning of the journey, the ship is well-stocked with supplies — fresh food, clean water, and plenty of spare parts to fix anything that breaks. These supplies are stem cells, the body's master resources, responsible for replenishing and repairing the tissues that wear down over time. But as the voyage continues, those supplies begin to dwindle. The reserves of stem cells gradually dry up, and when something breaks, there's nothing left to fix it. This depletion is known as stem cell exhaustion.

~❧

## What Are Stem Cells?

Unlike regular cells, which have specific functions and limited lifespans, stem cells can divide and differentiate into new, specialized cells whenever the body needs them, allowing them to produce new cells that replace old, damaged, or dead ones.

Stem cells are the body's go-to repairmen, responsible for maintaining and replenishing tissues throughout our lives. Different types of stem cells are found in various parts of the body: some replenish blood cells, some maintain bones and connective tissues, and still others help regenerate parts of the nervous system.

Throughout our youth, stem cells are abundant and highly active, repairing everything from skin injuries to muscle damage. But as we age, the regenerative capacity of stem cells declines. They either become dysfunctional, stop dividing, or die off. This gradual depletion of stem cells contributes to the aging process and the onset of many age-related diseases.

~♪

## How Stem Cell Exhaustion Happens

One of the primary culprits of stem cell exhaustion is cellular damage. As stem cells divide throughout life, they accumulate mutations and damage from environmental factors like radiation or toxins, as well as from internal processes like oxidative stress. This damage can cause stem cells to enter a state of senescence, where they stop dividing and functioning altogether, or to undergo apoptosis (a type of cellular suicide). Over time, this reduces the pool of functional stem cells.

Telomere shortening is another major culprit. Just like other cells in the body, stem cells have telomeres—the protective caps at the ends of chromosomes that shorten with each cell division. As telomeres shorten, they signal the cell to stop dividing, which leads to stem cell exhaustion. This process is particularly critical in highly regenerative tissues like the skin, muscles, and blood, where stem cells are called upon to divide frequently throughout life.

Another significant mechanism is the disruption of stem cell niches. Stem cells rely on specialized environments, or "niches," to maintain their function. These niches provide the signals and support that stem cells need to thrive. But as we age, these niches themselves become dysfunctional, offering fewer supportive signals and instead contributing to inflammation and fibrosis.

~~❧~~

## The Impact on Aging and Disease

As the pool of functional stem cells dwindles, the body's ability to repair itself diminishes. This decline leads to a variety of age-related changes, from the thinning of skin to the weakening of muscles and bones. Stem cell exhaustion is particularly impactful in tissues that rely on high turnover rates, such as the blood and immune systems.

First, let's turn to the hematopoietic system. This is the body's blood-forming system, responsible for producing all the different types of blood cells — red blood cells, white blood cells, and platelets — that circulate throughout your body. This process, called hematopoiesis, takes place primarily in the bone marrow, a soft, spongy tissue found inside bones. Stem cell exhaustion in the hemapoietic system leads to a decrease in the production of blood cells, which can cause anemia and impair the immune response, known as "immunosenescence". This is why older adults are more prone to illnesses like the flu or pneumonia, and why recovery from infections takes longer. Immunosenescence also plays a role in the increased risk of cancer seen in older adults, as the immune system becomes less adept at detecting and destroying cancerous cells.

The musculoskeletal system, too, suffers from stem cell exhaustion. Here, the main players are mesenchymal stem cells, which are responsible for maintaining bones and connective tissues. Depletion of these stem cells contributes to the development of osteoporosis, causing the bones to become less dense and more fragile. This increases the risk of fractures, which can be life-threatening in older adults. Muscle stem cells are also depleted with age, leading to sarcopenia (the age-related loss of muscle mass and strength) and making it harder for individuals to stay active and independent.

In the nervous system, stem cell exhaustion in neural stem cells impairs the brain's ability to generate new neurons, which may contribute to cognitive decline and the development of neurodegenerative diseases such as Alzheimer's and Parkinson's. As the ability to replace damaged or dead neurons declines, the brain's overall function deteriorates, leading to memory loss, reduced cognitive abilities, and other symptoms associated with aging.

~~●

## Therapeutic Approaches to Combat Stem Cell Exhaustion

Research into combating stem cell exhaustion has opened new avenues in regenerative medicine. One promising approach is the use of induced pluripotent stem cells (iPSCs), which are adult cells reprogrammed to a stem-cell-like state. These iPSCs can theoretically be used to replenish stem cell pools in aging tissues, offering a potential avenue for regenerating damaged tissues without the ethical concerns associated with embryonic stem cells.

Another approach involves targeting senescent cells with drugs known as senolytics. By clearing out senescent cells, scientists hope to reduce inflammation and restore a healthier environment for stem cells to function. Early studies in animal models have shown that senolytic therapies can improve tissue function, reduce frailty, and extend lifespan.

Other experimental therapies focus on enhancing the function of existing stem cells. For example, NAD+ precursors, such as nicotinamide riboside (NR) and nicotinamide mononucleotide (NMN), have been shown to boost mitochondrial function in stem cells, potentially helping to delay the onset of exhaustion and restore some regenerative capacity.

# CHAPTER 12

# Altered Intercellular Communication: When Cells Stop Playing Nice

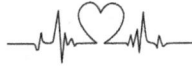

O ur bodies rely on a constant flow of messages between cells to function properly. This process, known as intercellular communication, ensures that cells coordinate activities, respond to changes, and maintain the body's overall health. With age, however, these communication channels begin to break down. Altered intercellular communication, one of the hallmarks of aging, describes how the signals between cells change over time, often leading to widespread dysfunction and contributing to diseases that we associate with growing older.

Just like static on a radio interrupts a clear signal, aging introduces disruptions in the ways cells talk to one another. Normally, cells send out chemical signals—like hormones, cytokines, and other molecules—to tell each other what to do. These messages ensure everything from tissue repair to immune responses happens smoothly. But as we age, these signals become distorted. In some cases, too many harmful signals are sent out, while beneficial communication diminishes. The result is a body that's out of sync, where the breakdown in communication amplifies aging itself.

## How Intercellular Communication Changes with Age

One of the most prominent changes in intercellular communication as we age is the rise of inflammation—specifically chronic inflammation. This isn't the useful, short-term inflammation that helps heal wounds or fight infections, but rather a persistent, low-grade inflammation that affects tissues over the long term. Senescent cells—cells that have stopped dividing but refuse to die—are major culprits in this. They release harmful substances into the environment, which encourages surrounding cells to enter a similar dysfunctional state. These signals lead to tissue damage, reduced immune function, and contribute to the onset of various age-related conditions like heart disease, arthritis, and diabetes.

But inflammation isn't the only issue. As we age, the hormonal balance within our body shifts. In younger years, hormones regulate everything from growth to metabolism, but aging alters this delicate balance. For example, certain hormonal signals that once promoted tissue maintenance, like growth factors, decline, leaving tissues unable to repair themselves as efficiently. At the same time, pro-aging factors—like *nuclear factor kappa B (NF-kB)*, a protein complex involved in inflammatory responses—become more active. This imbalance accelerates tissue deterioration.

~๑

## The Role of the Immune System

Another key player in altered intercellular communication is the immune system, which becomes less efficient with age. Immune cells normally communicate with each other to detect and destroy harmful invaders like bacteria or viruses. But this communication falters as we grow older, leading to a weakened immune response. Older immune cells can release the wrong signals, contributing to immunosenescence, where the immune system loses its ability to effectively fight infections. Complicating matters, the inflammatory signals from senescent cells cause immune cells to mistakenly attack healthy tissues, further compounding the damage.

This breakdown of immune communication also contributes to autoimmune diseases, where the immune system begins attacking the body's own cells. This is why older adults are more likely to experience conditions like rheumatoid arthritis or type 2 diabetes, which are linked to both chronic inflammation and immune miscommunication.

~

## Diseases Linked to Altered Intercellular Communication

The disruption of intercellular communication isn't just a biological inconvenience—it's directly tied to many diseases of aging. One of the most obvious impacts is on cardiovascular health. Chronic inflammation from altered signaling contributes to the buildup of atherosclerotic plaques in the arteries, which can lead to heart attacks and strokes. Similarly, this pro-inflammatory environment is a major driver of neurodegenerative diseases like Alzheimer's and Parkinson's, where the brain's cells receive damaged or distorted signals, leading to cognitive decline

Beyond inflammation, aging also affects the endocrine system, the network of glands that release hormones. As hormonal communication breaks down, it contributes to metabolic diseases like type 2 diabetes and osteoporosis. For example, insulin signaling becomes less effective with age, making it harder for the body to regulate blood sugar levels. Similarly, changes in hormone levels can lead to weakened bones, increasing the risk of fractures and falls

~~

## Fighting Back: Potential Interventions

Understanding how altered intercellular communication drives aging has opened the door to potential therapies aimed at restoring healthy signaling. One area of research is focused on reducing chronic inflammation, with drugs targeting the pathways that amplify pro-inflammatory signals. Senolytics, drugs that selectively kill senescent cells, have shown promise in reducing the harmful effects of SASP, thereby decreasing inflammation and improving tissue function

Another intriguing area of research is parabiosis, a process where the circulatory systems of young and old animals are connected. Studies in mice have shown that exposing older animals to the blood of younger ones can reverse some signs of aging, likely by diluting harmful pro-aging factors present in older blood. While still far from being a feasible treatment for humans, this research highlights the importance of addressing age-related changes in bloodborne signals

# CHAPTER 13

# Chronic Inflammation: The Body's Slow-Burning Fire

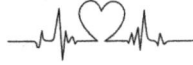

―√√⌒2√√―

Imagine inflammation as a fire within the body. When it's a controlled blaze, it serves a purpose, helping clear out infections or heal injuries. But in aging, this once-beneficial response becomes a smoldering flame, no longer fighting off infections but instead stoking the fires of aging itself. This is how chronic inflammation, or "inflammaging," operates: a low-grade, persistent state of immune activity that gradually wears down tissues, accelerates aging, and leaves the body vulnerable to disease.

Inflammation normally kicks in when immune cells send out chemical signals—like cytokines and other immune molecules—that draw resources to areas that need repair or protection. But with age, these signals start to backfire. Cells can overproduce inflammatory molecules, while immune cells lose their ability to tell the difference between harmful and healthy cells, leading to unintended damage.

~୬

## Mechanisms of Inflammaging: The Pathways of Chronic Inflammation

A major culprit behind chronic inflammation is the decline in immune system efficiency. The immune system has a finely tuned balance between activation and suppression. Yet as we age, this balance is thrown askew, causing the system to become overactive in some ways and underactive in others. Overactive immune cells release inflammatory signals that heighten inflammaging, while underactive responses fail to clear damaged cells effectively. This imbalance increases vulnerability to infections and perpetuates low-level inflammation throughout the body, leaving the immune system in a constant state of "red alert."

At a cellular level, one of the main drivers of inflammaging is a pathway called *cGAS-STING*, which senses damaged DNA and responds by igniting inflammatory responses. When things are running as they should, cGAS-STING plays a protective role, identifying and attacking cells that may be cancerous or infected. With time, however, this system becomes overactive, mistaking harmless cells for threats and sparking inflammation throughout the body. Indeed, animal models suggest that blocking cGAS-STING reduces chronic inflammation, pointing to its pivotal role in aging and inflammation management.

Another influential player is *NF-kB*, a protein complex involved in regulating immune responses. As cells age, oxidative stress, DNA damage, and metabolic shifts trigger NF-kB to increase the production of inflammatory molecules. Instead of coordinating precise responses to infections or injuries, NF-kB promotes the kind of widespread inflammation associated with chronic diseases. These pathways don't work alone; instead, they interact in ways that amplify one another, creating a feedback loop that perpetuates inflammation across tissues and organs as we age.

Mitochondrial dysfunction also contributes significantly to inflammaging. Mitochondria are central to controlled cell death, or apoptosis, through a process called mitochondrial outer membrane permeabilization (MOMP). MOMP helps remove damaged cells while limiting immune responses. However, senescent cells experience a low-level, "minority" form of MOMP (miMOMP), which keeps them in a limbo between life and death. This partial permeabilization prevents their breakdown, allowing them to continuously release inflammatory signals that add to the chronic inflammation associated with aging. Blocking MOMP in these cells has shown potential to reduce inflammation, pointing toward new therapeutic strategies aimed at mitigating inflammaging and improving overall health.

## Diseases Associated with Chronic Inflammation

Chronic inflammation plays a pivotal role in many age-related diseases. For instance, in cardiovascular disease, inflammation destabilizes the lining of blood vessels. Inflammatory cells, like macrophages, infiltrate the vessel walls and release enzymes and reactive oxygen species (ROS) that oxidize low-density lipoproteins (LDL), a type of cholesterol. These modified LDL molecules accumulate within the vessel walls, attracting more immune cells and forming fatty plaques. Over time, these plaques harden, narrow the arteries, and restrict blood flow—a condition known as atherosclerosis. Chronic inflammation also weakens the structural integrity of these plaques, increasing the likelihood that they will rupture, leading to clots that can cause heart attacks or strokes.

In neurodegenerative diseases, like Alzheimer's and Parkinson's, chronic inflammation disrupts normal cell signaling in the brain, contributing to cognitive decline and neuron death. Microglia, the brain's resident immune cells, become overactive and release inflammatory cytokines, which can trigger a cascade of damaging events. These cytokines encourage the formation and spread of protein aggregates, such as amyloid-beta plaques and tau tangles in Alzheimer's, that interfere with neural function and connectivity. Furthermore, this environment causes the blood-brain barrier to become more permeable, allowing harmful molecules to enter the brain and amplify the inflammatory response, progressively accelerating neuronal damage.

In metabolic diseases like type 2 diabetes, chronic inflammation interferes with the cells' ability to respond to insulin, a hormone that regulates glucose uptake. Pro-inflammatory cytokines, released from fat cells (particularly in abdominal obesity), impair the signaling pathways involved in insulin's actions on cells. One key pathway affected is the insulin receptor substrate (IRS) pathway, where cytokines induce serine phosphorylation of IRS proteins, inhibiting insulin signaling and leading to insulin resistance. This disrupts glucose homeostasis, causing blood sugar levels to remain elevated and eventually leading to systemic metabolic disturbances, including further inflammation, oxidative stress, and complications like kidney disease.

# CHAPTER 14

# Dysbiosis: When the Body's Microbial Ecosystem Falls Out of Balance

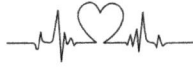

—√∿♡2∿√—

O ur body harbors trillions of microbes, collectively called the microbiome, which play a critical role in digestion, immune function, and even mental health. The gut microbiome, in particular, helps break down food, produce essential vitamins, and maintain the integrity of the gut lining, acting as a protective barrier between the outside world and our internal organs. But as we age, this microbial community changes. The diversity of beneficial microbes declines, and harmful or inflammatory bacteria begin to thrive. This imbalance is what we call dysbiosis, and it is closely linked to the aging process and the progression of age-related diseases.

～♪

## How Dysbiosis Develops with Age

Aging brings changes to nearly every system in the body, and the gut is no exception. For example, the slowing down of gastrointestinal motility (the movement of food through the digestive tract) creates conditions where certain bacteria can overgrow. We also start to produce less stomach acid as we grow older, allowing bacteria that would normally be killed to survive and multiply. Over time, these changes shift the composition of the microbiome, reducing the population of beneficial microbes while promoting the growth of potentially harmful ones.

Another factor contributing to dysbiosis in aging is the immune system's declining efficiency. The immune system normally keeps harmful microbes in check, but as it weakens with age, its ability to regulate the microbiome falters. This weakened immune surveillance allows pathogenic bacteria to establish a stronger foothold, creating an environment ripe for dysbiosis. Age-related inflammation worsens this imbalance, as inflammation in the gut further disrupts the microbial environment.

~•

## Mechanisms Behind Dysbiosis

The mechanisms driving dysbiosis are complex and interconnected, often involving a feedback loop between microbial imbalances and bodily inflammation. When beneficial bacteria decrease, the byproducts they produce, like short-chain fatty acids (SCFAs), also diminish. SCFAs, such as butyrate, play a crucial role in gut health by nourishing colon cells and reducing inflammation. With fewer SCFAs, the gut lining becomes more susceptible to damage, and the immune system's inflammatory response kicks in, aggravating the existing microbial imbalance.

The breakdown of the gut barrier function is another key mechanism of dysbiosis. In a healthy gut, the lining acts like a highly selective gatekeeper, allowing nutrients in while keeping harmful substances out. Dysbiosis can weaken this barrier, making it more permeable—a condition often referred to as "leaky gut." When the gut lining is compromised, toxins, bacteria, and undigested food particles can leak into the bloodstream, triggering systemic inflammation. This inflammation then exacerbates dysbiosis, creating a self-perpetuating cycle that impacts the body beyond the gut, increasing vulnerability to diseases.

~●

## Diseases Associated with Dysbiosis

The effects of dysbiosis extend far beyond gastrointestinal discomfort. Research has linked dysbiosis to a range of diseases, particularly those associated with aging. For instance, cardiovascular disease is influenced by the microbiome. Certain gut bacteria produce trimethylamine-N-oxide (TMAO) when they metabolize foods rich in choline and carnitine, like red meat and eggs. Elevated levels of TMAO in the blood are associated with an increased risk of atherosclerosis, the hardening and narrowing of arteries that can lead to heart attacks and strokes.

In the realm of neurodegenerative diseases, dysbiosis has been implicated in conditions like Alzheimer's and Parkinson's disease. The gut-brain axis—a bidirectional communication system between the gut and the brain—is influenced heavily by the microbiome. An imbalance in gut bacteria can disrupt this communication, leading to increased inflammation that affects brain health. In Alzheimer's disease, inflammatory molecules from the gut can travel through the bloodstream, contributing to neuroinflammation and the accumulation of amyloid plaques in the brain.

Dysbiosis also plays a role in metabolic disorders like type 2 diabetes. The microbial imbalance disrupts insulin sensitivity by influencing fat storage and glucose metabolism. Inflammation triggered by dysbiosis affects insulin signaling pathways, leading to insulin resistance—a hallmark of type 2 diabetes. Furthermore, dysbiosis can contribute to obesity by increasing energy extraction from food, meaning that even without a change in diet, an altered microbiome can cause weight gain.

~❧

## Tackling Dysbiosis: Potential Therapies

Understanding dysbiosis and its role in aging has led to a growing interest in therapies that restore a healthy microbiome balance. Probiotics—live beneficial bacteria—are commonly used to replenish the gut with beneficial microbes. While probiotics can help, they often have a limited and temporary effect. Prebiotics, which are fibers that feed beneficial bacteria, can be combined with probiotics to promote the growth of these beneficial microbes and improve gut health over time.

Another approach is fecal microbiota transplantation (FMT), where microbiota from a healthy donor is transplanted into the gut of a patient to restore microbial balance. Though still in experimental stages for many conditions, FMT has shown promise in treating infections like Clostridium difficile and is being investigated for its potential in addressing dysbiosis-related diseases in older adults.

# PART II
# What Can *You* Do?

Now that we've covered the fundamental mechanisms governing the aging process, it's time to start asking the pressing questions: What does this mean for *me*? Is there anything *I* can do?

It's well and good to understand aging in the abstract, but in the end, the reason we care about it is exceedingly concrete: it robs us of time spent in good health, doing the things we love. It's only natural to wonder if we might not be able to steal some of that time back for ourselves.

That's exactly what this section is about: actionable steps that you can take to improve your chances at living a longer, healthier life. The goal is plain to see, we want to remain "biologically young" even when we are chronologically old. That is, we want to stave off the usual symptoms of aging as long as we possibly can.

Easier said than done.

But we aren't completely in the dark. Over the past few decades, scientists have amassed a wealth of new research on topics in longevity studies. While a big chunk of this research focuses on potential new "anti-aging" drugs, a portion also deals with what we might call "lifestyle factors." These include the usual, boring suspects: diet, exercise, sleep, stress, and so on. Tedious as they may be, the scientific literature consistently highlights the importance of these factors in shaping long — and healthy! — lives. So, while we all want that elixir of youth, many of the most effective strategies currently available are in *your* hands. They aren't necessarily quick, nor are they necessarily the easiest, but they do pay off, as evidenced by study after study.

# CHAPTER 15

# A Shift in Perspective: Prevention over Treatment

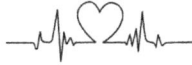

We've all heard it before, "an ounce of prevention is worth a pound of cure." It has solidified itself as one of those idioms that gets thrown around in conversations on health and well being. The annoying thing about clichés is that, more often than not, they have something going for them. They stick around because, well, they *do* convey crucial nuggets of wisdom. This one is no different.

While we are all implicitly aware of the power of prevention, it often gets lost in the noise of everyday life. This is especially true given how little most healthcare systems emphasize preventative care — here in the U.S., ours is very much a system built around treatment. One quick glance at the way we address diet makes that beyond obvious. Unhealthy diets are a major driver of illness, from heart disease, diabetes, obesity, all the way to mental health issues like depression and anxiety. In fact, diet-related illnesses are now the leading cause of death in the U.S., responsible for more fatalities than smoking. And the financial toll? Enormous. Treating conditions like high blood pressure, diabetes, and high cholesterol currently costs around $400 billion each year. Within the next 25 years, that number is expected to soar to a staggering $1.3 trillion.

Despite this, a 2023 survey of over 1,000 U.S. medical students revealed a troubling gap in nutrition education: 58% reported receiving no formal training, and those who did averaged just three hours per year—falling far short of the 25 hours recommended back in 1985 by the U.S. Committee on Nutrition in Medical Education. Recent studies show this issue is worsening, with only 7.8% of students in 2023 reporting 20 or more hours of nutrition education across all four years of med school, despite various government efforts to address the shortfall.

The effects are clear. In one assessment of nutrition knowledge, more than half of 250 first- and second-year medical students failed, even though 55% had felt confident advising patients on nutrition. And this gap is not limited to the U.S.; a 2018 global study confirmed that insufficient nutrition training for medical students is a widespread issue, leaving future doctors around the world underprepared to counsel patients on one of the most fundamental aspects of health.

All this talk about prevention, but does it *really* matter? Yes. A lot, in fact. How do we know? By studying the pioneers of longevity, "centenarians." Centenarians are people who have reached the age of 100 (or older). A study published in August of 2024 managed to answer a lingering question about these super agers: do they reach 100 by surviving, delaying, or avoiding diseases?

The study looked at 170,800 individuals born between 1912 and 1922 in Stockholm County, Sweden. Of these, only 1.4% —2367 people— lived to be 100 years old, with most of the others passing away in their eighties.

To get a sense of what separated the centenarians from their shorter-lived peers, the team of researchers used historical data to keep track of the cohort from 1972 to 2022. This allowed them to compare everyone's health starting at age 60 onwards, giving them a richer understanding of the ways centenarians compare to their peers at various stages of life.

The findings were crystal clear: centenarians tended to reach their advanced age not by being more resilient to diseases, but by delaying the onset of diseases in the first place. That is, they avoid diseases — especially those chronic diseases that we constantly hear about (heart disease, type 2 diabetes, high blood pressure, etc.). Crucially, this remained the case at every age, not just in youth. And even at the age of 100, centenarians had still not caught up to the disease risks that individuals who die at earlier ages exhibited.

These results aren't confined to this one study either; there are a number of others, from around the globe, that point in the same direction. For example, a Danish study explored the aging patterns of those born in 1905, discovering that individuals who reached 100 years of age tended to have fewer hospital visits and shorter hospital stays compared to those who passed away younger. Findings from Okinawa—famed for its supercentenarians— echo this observation, revealing that most people in this elite age group experience minimal or no significant diseases until they hit a century. Remarkably, conditions like coronary heart disease and stroke were exceptionally uncommon among them before reaching 100, lending more weight to the resilience displayed by those who live longest. And in Spain, again, centenarians generally experience fewer health problems and need less medical care —both in hospitals and through primary doctors— compared to people in their 80s and 90s, hinting that those who live to 100 often enjoy better overall health.

To live a long, healthy life you need to avoid disease. What could be more obvious. And yet when we operate under a treatment-forward framework, the emphasis is not on disease avoidance. Instead, the underlying assumption is that "if I get sick, I'll get treated and recover." As these centenarian studies suggest, the key is to be proactive, to maintain good health from the get go. Think of it like interest rates on savings, the money you make early on pays off double later on. Healthy living in early life extends to later life.

# CHAPTER 16

# Medical Advice from the Ancients?

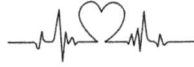

Our fixation with eternal living is by no means new. From temples to religions to potions, our ancestors have long been obsessed with the same question. The pyramids in Egypt are perhaps the most obvious example of such endeavors. They were monuments that sought to help pharaohs extend their life "beyond life" — death, in this case, would be nothing more than the beginning of another life. While pacifying, this approach isn't exactly what most of us have in mind when we think of longevity.

The Chinese emperor Qin Shihuang, known as "the first emperor of China" for having unified all of the warring states, opted for a more direct line of attack: he ordered his court physicians to make him immortal. Indeed, he even sent a minister on a mission to find a mythical elixir of immortality. Unsurprisingly, this minister never returned; showing up empty handed would not have played out well, and showing up with a fake elixir wouldn't have been much better.

But Qin Shihuang's local physicians concocted potions with mercury, a toxic metal that can lead to all kinds of nasty issues: memory problems, skin rashes, trouble seeing, poor coordination, trouble hearing, muscle weakness, numbness in the hands and feet, anxiety, or trouble speaking. In severe cases, mercury poisoning can cause kidney problems, a drop in intelligence, and even death — so much for an "elixir of immortality". Rather than aid his pursuit of eternal life, the elixir he drank likely shortened his lifespan, contributing to his death at the ripe old age of 49.[1]

The emperor's tomb, a massive complex famed for the terracotta soldiers guarding over it, has been shown to emit high levels of atmospheric mercury compared to the surrounding environment. The soil around the tomb is also noticeably higher in mercury than usual. Perhaps this was Qin Shihuang's final attempt at securing immortality? We likely won't find out anytime soon, as the tomb has remained sealed since its completion nearly 2000 years ago, with no plans to open it (archaeologists worry that opening the tomb will jeopardize its contents).

While the above examples are rather extreme, most cultures also had more practical medical advice, some of which is shockingly similar to what you might expect to see if you picked up a contemporary fitness magazine.

If we pan westwards for a moment, we can take a look at some of the lifestyle tips offered up by the Greeks and Romans. What stands out is their recognition that the secret to a long, fulfilling life isn't found in fleeting efforts or miracle cures — it is in the art of daily living. Figures like Gorgias of Leontini, who reportedly lived beyond 100 years, knew this well. Gorgias once quipped that his secret to longevity lay in avoiding actions driven solely by pleasure or

---

[1] It should be noted that there is debate about this account of events, with some scholars casting doubt on the veracity of the claims. Expert archaeologist Duan Qingbo, for example, argues that the use of liquid mercury in elixirs wasn't popularized until the later Han dynasty (which succeeded Qin's rule). Regardless, it is clear that mercury was at one point or another used as a primary ingredient in elixirs aimed at bestowing immortality.

obligation, a cheeky yet profound nod to the power of balance and moderation.

This philosophy wasn't just talk; it was reflected in the lives of many prominent figures. Titus Vestricius Spurinna, a Roman senator, followed a carefully structured routine even into his seventies. Every morning, he'd set off on a three-mile walk, followed by activities like ball games, sunbathing, and listening to light readings. His afternoons were no less deliberate, balancing physical exertion with leisure and intellectual stimulation. Spurinna's life was a testament to the ancients' belief in harmony — a dance between movement and rest, effort and relaxation.

For Roman physician Aulus Cornelius Celsus, the key to staying youthful lay in variety. He advised alternating between the countryside and the city, taking up invigorating activities like sailing or hunting, and keeping both the body and mind active. To Celsus, inactivity was the great accelerator of aging, while deliberate physical effort slowed its relentless march. Even simple practices, like walking or reading aloud, were seen as powerful tools to maintain vitality. Celsus' recommendations weren't just about avoiding disease — they were about embracing life fully, no matter one's age.

Galen, one of the most influential physicians of antiquity, had little patience for poor lifestyle choices. He believed that many ailments arose from overindulgence, inactivity, and stress — problems that sound all too familiar today. Galen admired the disciplined habits of his colleague, Antiochus, who maintained an active lifestyle and a simple, nourishing diet well into his eighties. Bread, honey, and lightly prepared meats made up the core of Antiochus' meals, proving that health didn't require extravagance, just consistency and care.

The Greeks and Romans understood something profound about the human experience: health isn't only about avoiding sickness, it's about living well. They remind us that longevity doesn't come from shortcuts or extremes but from the rhythm of everyday life. Their practices — walking, eating simply, finding joy in movement and rest — are as accessible today as they were thousands of years ago.

Indeed, the same advice holds true now as it did then, the only difference is that we have the scientific data to support it. Let's take a closer look.

# CHAPTER 17

# Exercise and Longevity

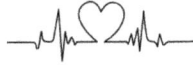

$—\!\!\backslash\!\!\vert\!\!\sim\!\!\heartsuit 2\!\!\backslash\!\!\vert\!\!\sim\!\!—$

In a world where sitting has become the default position — whether at desks, on couches, or in cars — the consequences for our health are profound. Even in countries like the Netherlands, known for their cycling culture and general activity levels, the creeping dominance of "chair-use disorder" is taking its toll.

Exercise offers a way to push back against this encroaching trend. At its core, physical activity initiates a cascade of biological signals that ripple across the body, touching every organ and system. It impacts aging not only by slowing the ticking of our biological clocks but by rewiring how our brains and bodies communicate — a cellular symphony powered by molecules like myokines (proteins released by muscles during exercise) and exerkines (proteins released by the rest of the body during exercise).

~●

## Rewiring the Brain and Body Connection

At a cellular level, physical activity triggers profound changes in the brain, fundamentally altering how neurons communicate and adapt. These changes not only improve cognitive function but also fortify the brain against the ravages of aging and disease. To understand how this happens, we need to explore the dialogue between muscles and the brain — a conversation powered by molecules like brain-derived neurotrophic factor (BDNF) and irisin.

Imagine your brain as a dense forest, with neurons as trees and their synaptic connections as sprawling root systems. Over time, without care and nurturing, some connections weaken, and the forest begins to thin — a process often associated with aging and cognitive decline. Exercise, however, acts like a rejuvenating rainstorm, promoting the growth of new neural pathways and strengthening existing ones. This process, known as neuroplasticity, is the brain's ability to rewire itself in response to new experiences, learning, or, in this case, physical activity.

At the heart of this transformation is BDNF, a protein often referred to as "fertilizer for the brain." When you exercise, particularly during aerobic or high-intensity workouts, your muscles and brain release signals that stimulate the production of BDNF. This protein supports the survival and growth of neurons, enhances synaptic connections, and improves overall brain health. Think of BDNF as a foreman overseeing the forest's restoration, ensuring new trees are planted and the roots of old ones are reinforced.

But the story doesn't end with BDNF. Another critical player in this muscle-brain dialogue is irisin, a hormone released during exercise that has garnered significant attention for its neuroprotective effects. Studies have shown that irisin can reduce levels of amyloid-beta plaques — sticky protein clumps that are hallmarks of Alzheimer's disease — by activating brain-supporting cells called astrocytes. Astrocytes, which act as the brain's custodians, respond to irisin by clearing away these harmful deposits and maintaining the brain's structural integrity. In essence, irisin serves as a messenger, traveling from the muscles to the brain to deliver instructions for repair and rejuvenation.

Exercise also stimulates "neurogenesis," a fancy term to describe the birth of new neurons. This is particularly noticeable in the hippocampus, which is a brain region crucial for learning and memory. For decades, scientists believed that humans were born with a fixed number of neurons, but more recent research suggests that neurogenesis can continue into old age — if we provide the right conditions. Exercise is one such condition. By enhancing blood flow to the brain and delivering a cocktail of beneficial molecules, physical activity creates an environment where new neurons can thrive.

For example, in aged individuals, high-intensity interval training (HIIT) has been shown to significantly improve hippocampal-dependent learning and memory. These findings underscore that, even late in life, the brain retains a remarkable capacity for growth and adaptation when spurred by exercise. Participants in these studies not only performed better on cognitive tests but also enjoyed measurable increases in brain volume — a striking reversal of the typical shrinkage associated with aging.

The connection between exercise and the brain isn't limited to direct molecular interactions. The physical act of moving also reduces inflammation in the brain, which plays a critical role in maintaining cognitive health. Chronic inflammation, often driven by aging and lifestyle factors, damages neurons and accelerates cognitive decline. Exercise dampens this inflammatory response by promoting the release of anti-inflammatory molecules like *clusterin*, a protein shown to reduce neuroinflammation and enhance memory. In this way, physical activity acts as both a shield and a repair mechanism, protecting the brain from harm while promoting its natural ability to heal.

What makes these findings particularly exciting is the holistic nature of the benefits. Exercise doesn't just work on one part of the brain or target a single pathway; it creates a network of improvements that reinforce one another. BDNF enhances neuroplasticity, irisin clears toxic proteins, neurogenesis replenishes the brain's cellular reserves, and anti-inflammatory signals ensure a hospitable environment for all these processes to occur. Together, they paint a picture of a brain that is not only more resistant to aging but also more capable of adapting to new challenges and retaining its vitality.

When all is said and done, regular physical activity could be one of the most accessible and effective tools for maintaining brain health and preventing cognitive decline. And the best part? It's never too late to start. Whether it's a brisk walk, a swim, or an intense workout session, every movement you make contributes to a cascade of benefits that extend far beyond the gym. By fostering a healthier brain, exercise helps ensure that you can not only live longer but live better, with sharper memories, quicker thinking, and a greater ability to engage with the world around you.

~❦

## Muscle Talk: The Language of Myokines and Exosomes

When we exercise, our muscles do far more than contract and relax — they transform into dynamic communication hubs, sending signals throughout the body to enhance function and resilience. These signals are delivered in the form of *myokines*, specialized proteins secreted by muscle cells, and *exosomes*, tiny vesicles carrying molecular instructions. This muscle-generated "language" is rewriting how we understand the benefits of physical activity, extending its influence well beyond muscle growth to support brain health, immune function, and overall vitality.

Unlike the brain's direct molecular connections, discussed above, the muscles use a more diffuse yet equally powerful network to communicate. Myokines are one of the key components of this network. Released during muscle contractions, they travel through the bloodstream to influence the behavior of distant organs. For example, *interleukin-6 (IL-6)*, a myokine that spikes during exercise, helps regulate inflammation and energy metabolism. While IL-6 is often associated with chronic inflammation when overproduced in unhealthy contexts, during exercise, it takes on an entirely different role — acting as a natural anti-inflammatory that helps reset the body's balance.

Then there are exosomes, microscopic delivery vehicles packed with proteins, lipids, and even genetic material. Unlike myokines, which act more like free-floating chemical messengers, exosomes operate with targeted precision. These vesicles are like microscopic delivery trucks, ferrying cargo from your muscles to distant organs such as your brain, liver, and even your gut. Once they arrive, exosomes release their payload, influencing cellular behavior in profound ways. For instance, exosomes have been shown to carry neurotrophic factors — proteins that promote the growth and survival of neurons. In essence, your muscles are delivering care packages to your brain, ensuring its health and resilience.

The communication network doesn't stop at the brain. Exercise-induced exosomes also impact metabolic health by delivering molecular cargo to the liver and other metabolic organs. This improves glucose metabolism, enhances insulin sensitivity, and reduces the risk of type 2 diabetes. Meanwhile, other exosomes target the gut microbiome, fostering a more balanced microbial environment that supports digestion, immunity, and even mental health.

One of the most exciting aspects of this muscle-driven signaling system is its adaptability. The type of exercise you perform shapes the molecules your muscles release. High-intensity interval training (HIIT), for example, might focus on releasing neuroprotective factors, while resistance training emphasizes molecules that repair and grow muscle fibers. This tailored response ensures that different forms of exercise can support the body in complementary ways, reinforcing the interconnectedness of muscle and systemic health.

For aging populations, the significance of these findings cannot be overstated. Skeletal muscles, often overlooked in discussions of longevity, emerge as key players in preserving not only physical strength but also cognitive resilience. By continuing to send out beneficial signals through myokines and exosomes, muscles contribute their own arsenal of protective molecules, reinforcing the body's defenses on multiple fronts.

～

## What About the Heart?

While we've talked about the brain and the muscles, at the heart of exercise's systemic effects is the cardiovascular system. Regular aerobic activity strengthens the heart muscle, enabling it to pump blood more efficiently and deliver oxygen and nutrients to tissues with greater precision. Over time, this reduces strain on the heart, lowers resting blood pressure, and decreases the risk of cardiovascular diseases such as atherosclerosis and heart failure.

Physical activity reduces arterial stiffness, a key marker of aging, by increasing the production of *nitric oxide*, a molecule that helps blood vessels relax and expand. This improves blood flow and reduces the likelihood of clot formation, a precursor to strokes and heart attacks. Exercise also moderates lipid metabolism, helping to lower LDL ("bad") cholesterol while raising HDL ("good") cholesterol, further reducing the risk of plaque buildup in arteries.

~~

## Boosting the Immune System

Exercise also gives the immune system a potent boost, enhancing its ability to fend off illness and repair damage. Moderate, regular physical activity increases the circulation of immune cells, such as natural killer cells and T-cells, which play a vital role in identifying and destroying pathogens and abnormal cells. This immune enhancement is especially important as we age since the immune system naturally weakens over time.

What's remarkable is that these immune benefits extend to scenarios where the immune system is under acute stress. For example, people who maintain regular physical activity recover more quickly from infections and experience fewer complications from conditions like the flu or pneumonia.

~~

## From Gym Gains to Gut Gains

Less obvious but equally important is exercise's impact on the gut microbiome — the community of trillions of microorganisms residing in the digestive tract. These microbes play an essential role in digestion, immune defense, and even mental health, influencing the production of neurotransmitters like serotonin. With age, the gut microbiome often becomes less diverse, favoring bacteria that promote inflammation and metabolic dysfunction. Exercise, however, can reverse these changes, cultivating a richer and more balanced microbial ecosystem.

Physical activity increases the abundance of beneficial bacteria, which produce *short-chain fatty acids (SCFAs)*. Short-chain fatty acids nourish the cells lining the gut, strengthen the gut barrier, and reduce inflammation throughout the body. By enhancing gut integrity, exercise helps prevent "leaky gut," a condition where harmful substances escape into the bloodstream and fuel systemic inflammation.

These microbiome shifts have far-reaching implications. Improved gut health is associated with improved metabolic regulation, lower risks of obesity and diabetes, and even reduced symptoms of depression and anxiety. In this way, the gut becomes a critical mediator of exercise's systemic benefits, translating physical activity into enhanced health outcomes across multiple domains.

## The Real "Potion of Youth"?

What does all of this mean for us as we age? It means that exercise is a prescription for longevity. With each session, you're not just working out, you're setting the stage for a healthier, more resilient future. Even modest increases in movement can yield profound benefits.

Maybe numbers will help put things into perspective. Data from over 40,000 Americans, aged 40 and older, suggests that if everyone achieved the activity levels of the top 25% of the population, their life expectancy would increase by an average of 5.3 years. The impact is even more marked for those who are least active: for every added hour of walking each day, they could enjoy an extra six hours of life expectancy.

Any time you workout, you are sending a message from your muscles to the rest of your body: "Let's keep going." So lace up those shoes, because the benefits of movement extend far beyond the gym.

# CHAPTER 18

# Nutritional Approaches: Longevity Diets, Caloric Restriction, and Fasting

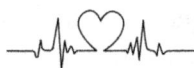

—⎁♡⎁—

The choices we make at mealtime ripple through our lives in ways we might not immediately see. Picture your diet as the foundation of a house — solid, balanced choices create a structure that stands strong against the storms of time, while poor habits leave it vulnerable to cracks and collapse. Luckily, the burgeoning field of nutritional geroscience is helping to make it clearer how what we eat — and just as crucially, when we eat — can profoundly impact the aging process. By tuning into this intricate symphony of nutrients and timing, we may unlock strategies to not only add years to our lives but also life to our years.

～

## Fasting and Caloric Restriction: Peering Beneath the Hood

Caloric restriction and intermittent fasting have emerged as two of the most intriguing dietary interventions for promoting longevity. Both involve cycles of energy deficit —caloric restriction entails a sustained reduction in calorie intake without malnutrition, while intermittent fasting alternates periods of eating with fasting. But what's happening beneath the surface when we limit calories or go without food for extended periods?

When the body detects a shortage of energy, it shifts into a kind of survival mode, triggering cellular responses designed to enhance efficiency and repair damage. At the heart of these benefits is autophagy, a cellular housekeeping process that clears out damaged proteins and organelles. As a quick refresher — it's been a while since our discussion on the hallmarks of aging — autophagy acts like a molecular recycling program, repurposing dysfunctional components to keep cells functioning optimally. This is especially important as we age, where cellular "trash" accumulates and contributes to diseases like Alzheimer's and Parkinson's.

Ketone bodies, produced during fasting, caloric restriction, or ketogenic diets, are particularly interesting in this regard. These molecules act as an alternative energy source for the brain when glucose levels drop. But beyond fueling brain cells, these molecules also appear to play a critical role in clearing damaged proteins. In studies conducted on mouse models, researchers observed that ketone bodies enhanced the brain's natural protein-clearing mechanisms. Specifically, a ketone body called *beta-hydroxybutyrate (BHB)* binds directly to misfolded proteins, increasing their solubility and making it easier for them to be removed by the brain's waste-management forces. This effect could explain why ketogenic diets and fasting protocols have shown promise in alleviating symptoms in neurodegenerative disorders — and, luckily for us, ketone bodies are easy to manipulate, making them a promising target for future drug development.

Fasting and caloric restriction also stimulate *mitochondrial biogenesis*, the production of new, more efficient mitochondria. These cellular powerhouses are responsible for generating the energy that fuels almost every bodily process. Over time, as mitochondria become less efficient, their dysfunction contributes to cellular aging and inflammation. By encouraging the replacement of old mitochondria with new ones, these dietary approaches help rejuvenate cells at a fundamental level.

A key player in these processes is the activation of *AMPK (AMP-activated protein kinase)*, an enzyme that acts as a cellular energy sensor. When energy levels dip, AMPK springs into action, enhancing fat metabolism, increasing insulin sensitivity, and improving glucose uptake. This metabolic recalibration has profound implications for reducing the risk of diseases like type 2 diabetes and metabolic syndrome.

Additionally, fasting and caloric restriction can influence the *epigenome*, the chemical modifications that regulate gene expression. By "turning on" genes associated with repair and longevity and "turning off" those linked to inflammation and damage, these interventions may partially "reprogram" cells to behave in a more youthful manner. Imagine fasting as a reset button for your genetic software, restoring the body's systems to a state of greater efficiency and resilience.

As it turns out, you may not even have to fully commit to fasting to enjoy the benefits. A recent study explored what they called the "fasting-mimicking diet (FMD)", a low-calorie, plant-based regimen designed to mimic fasting's benefits without complete food deprivation. Over just three cycles of the diet, participants experienced markers of reduced biological age, including decreased insulin resistance, lower levels of inflammatory cytokines, and improved liver health. This tells us that periodic dietary interventions can act as a metabolic reset, promoting longevity pathways and potentially delaying the onset of chronic diseases.

But few things are without complications. While the regenerative effects of fasting and caloric restriction are remarkable, there are some risks: prolonged or extreme caloric restriction can lead to a state of chronic energy deficiency, impairing immune function and increasing susceptibility to infections. In some cases, this can even accelerate muscle loss — a critical concern for aging populations where maintaining strength and mobility is key to boosting time spent in good health. So, although the body thrives on cycles of stress and recovery, overburdening it with prolonged calorie restriction may tip the scales toward harm rather than healing.

## The Hidden Costs of Ultra-Processed Foods

At the other end of the spectrum lies the modern diet, dominated by ultra-processed foods and high-calorie, low-nutrient options. These foods are engineered for taste and convenience, often at the expense of nutrition. While they might satisfy immediate cravings, their long-term effects on the body are far from benign. In the United Kingdom alone, for example, unhealthy diets are estimated to cause more than 75,000 premature deaths each year, including almost 17,000 deaths in the age group 15–70 years.

One of the primary issues with ultra-processed foods is their impact on the gut microbiome, the diverse community of microorganisms residing in our digestive system. These foods are often low in fiber and rich in additives, which can disrupt the balance of gut bacteria. Beneficial microbes thrive on fiber-rich diets, producing *short-chain fatty acids (SCFAs)* that strengthen the gut barrier and reduce inflammation. Without this support, harmful bacteria can proliferate, leading to "leaky gut," where toxins and inflammatory compounds enter the bloodstream.

Beyond the microbiome, the high sugar content of many processed foods creates a metabolic storm, causing spikes in blood glucose and insulin levels. Over time, this contributes to insulin resistance, a precursor to type 2 diabetes. Additionally, many ultra-processed foods contain *advanced glycation end products (AGEs)*, harmful compounds formed when sugars react with proteins or fats during cooking at high temperatures. AGEs accumulate in tissues, promoting oxidative stress and inflammation — key drivers of aging and chronic disease.

Perhaps most insidious is how these foods fuel chronic, low-grade inflammation. This persistent state of immune activation accelerates cellular damage and underlies many age-related conditions, from arthritis to cardiovascular disease. By constantly sounding the immune system's alarm bells, ultra-processed foods create a vicious cycle of damage and repair that hastens the aging process.

~♪

## Longevity Diets: Eating for a Better Future

In stark contrast, longevity diets emphasize nutrient-dense, minimally processed foods that nourish the body without overburdening it. These diets prioritize whole grains, fresh vegetables, nuts, legumes, and healthy fats, such as those found in olive oil and avocados. The Mediterranean diet is perhaps the best-known example of a longevity diet. Its emphasis on fresh, unprocessed foods and healthy fats has been linked to lower rates of heart disease, cancer, and neurodegenerative disorders.

This isn't empty rhetoric: we now know about proteomic signatures — molecular "footprints" in our blood — that correlate with adherence to these diets and predict reduced risks of diseases like diabetes and cardiovascular conditions. Every bite etches a biochemical signature, shaping our health trajectory at the cellular level.

A massive study from 2023 took a look at the dietary habits of almost 500,000 Britons to get a sense of just how big of a difference eating healthier can make. They found that individuals who transitioned from unhealthy eating habits to the Eatwell Guide dietary recommendations —a guide that shows you how much of what you eat should come from each food group— gained an additional 8.9 years of life expectancy for men and 8.6 years for women by age 40. And those that adopted actual longevity-focused dietary patterns, rich in nutrient-dense and minimally processed foods, were rewarded with life expectancy increases of more than a decade (for both men and women in the same population). Let me reiterate: A decade. Ten years. 3,650 extra days of laughter, love, and experiences — all potentially unlocked by the choices you make at mealtime.

Another exciting aspect of longevity diets is their ability to mimic some of the benefits of fasting and caloric restriction. Certain compounds in plant-based foods, such as *polyphenols* and *spermidine*, activate similar cellular pathways associated with repair and autophagy. For instance, spermidine —a compound found in foods like wheat germ, soybeans, and mushrooms— has been shown to promote cellular renewal and reduce inflammation, mimicking the effects of caloric restriction without requiring a drastic reduction in food intake. This is great news for those of us that struggle with the hunger pangs associated with fasting; you don't need to hold yourself back, you just need to change what you eat.

~⁙

## A Path Forward

The science of nutritional longevity is still unfolding, but its message is clear: what we eat and how we eat hold incredible power over the aging process. From fasting to carefully crafted diets, these interventions offer tools to not just extend life but improve its quality. By understanding the mechanisms at play —how food influences cellular repair, inflammation, and metabolism— we can make informed choices that align with our health goals.

The future promises a proliferation of personalized approaches, where diets are tailored to individual genetic profiles and circadian rhythms. But even today —and I know you are going to sigh because you've heard it a thousand times already— the steps are quite simple: eat whole foods, prioritize plant-based nutrients, and practice mindful eating patterns. Yes, it really can be that easy.

# CHAPTER 19

# Sleep and Aging: The Silent Regulator of Longevity

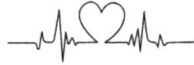

—⎯⎯ᴧᴧᴧ♡2ᴧᴧᴧ⎯⎯—

Imagine sleep as the body's nightly maintenance shift — a time when vital systems undergo repair, rejuvenation, and recalibration. Without this crucial downtime, it's like asking a factory to operate 24/7 without ever servicing the machinery; inefficiencies and breakdowns are inevitable. Emerging research continues to illuminate just how indispensable sleep is, not only for feeling refreshed but for maintaining robust physical health at the cellular and systemic levels.

~∘

## The Crucial Role of Sleep in Physical Health

At the forefront of this discovery is the "glymphatic system", the brain's waste disposal network, which relies heavily on quality sleep to function optimally. Think of this system as a cleaning crew, flushing out neurotoxic waste products like beta-amyloid and tau proteins, both associated with Alzheimer's disease. These proteins accumulate in the spaces between brain cells during the day, a natural byproduct of the brain's activity. During deep, non-REM sleep, rhythmic brain waves orchestrate the glymphatic system's action, driving cerebrospinal fluid (CSF) through the brain to transport these harmful substances out of the central nervous system.

This process hinges on synchronized neuronal oscillations — slow, rhythmic waves that sweep through the brain during sleep. These waves act like a hydraulic pump, facilitating the exchange of cerebrospinal and interstitial fluids and enhancing molecular clearance. Chronic sleep deprivation, however, significantly impairs glymphatic function, leaving waste to accumulate and increasing the risk of neurodegenerative diseases.

Sleep isn't just about safeguarding the brain, it has profound effects on the cardiovascular system as well. During sleep, blood pressure naturally dips, a phenomenon known as "nocturnal dipping," which allows the cardiovascular system to rest and recover. This nightly reprieve reduces strain on the heart and blood vessels, lowering the risk of hypertension and heart disease. Conversely, insufficient sleep disrupts this rhythm, leading to sustained high blood pressure and heightened risk of atherosclerosis — a condition I've already mentioned a few times, where arteries stiffen and clog with plaque.

Sleep also plays a pivotal role in immune defense. During deep sleep, the body ramps up the production of cytokines. These are proteins that regulate immune responses and help the body fight infections and inflammation. A single night of poor sleep can reduce T-cell activity, impair immune function, and even blunt the effectiveness of vaccines. Over time, chronic sleep deprivation weakens the immune system, leaving individuals more susceptible to illnesses.

And there's still more: sleep exerts a powerful influence on metabolic health too. While we sleep, the balance of hunger-regulating hormones —ghrelin and leptin— is restored. Ghrelin, which stimulates appetite, decreases, while leptin, the hormone signaling fullness, increases. Chronic sleep deprivation flips this balance, elevating ghrelin levels and suppressing leptin, often leading to overeating and weight gain. Over time, this imbalance contributes to obesity, insulin resistance, and an elevated risk of type 2 diabetes.

Similarly, sleep deprivation jumbles the brain's reward systems in such a way that calorie-dense, high-fat foods become irresistibly appealing. This means the increased attraction to unhealthy foods is not merely hormonal, it's "hedonic," a term to describe behaviours that are rooted in how the brain evaluates reward. Neuroimaging studies have pinpointed upregulated activity in the amygdala and hypothalamus, key regions involved in food motivation, after even a single night of poor sleep.

Finally, sleep is involved in cellular repair and regeneration. The production of *growth hormone*, which peaks during deep sleep, stimulates protein synthesis and aids in the recovery of muscles and tissues damaged during daily activities. This process is especially vital for athletes seeking recovery and for older adults aiming to preserve muscle mass and tissue integrity as they age.

~₰

## Cognitive Function and Mental Health

The importance of sleep isn't limited to the body, either. In fact, sleep is critical to maintaining our cognitive sharpness and emotional well-being. Its effects are profound, influencing how we think, learn, and feel daily. It's no surprise, then, that sleep is emerging as a key player in a number of processes, from consolidating memories to managing emotions and maintaining overall mental health.

During sleep, the brain organizes and solidifies information gathered throughout the day, transferring important memories to long-term storage. This process, known as memory consolidation, is fundamental for learning and adapting to new challenges.

On the flip side, chronic sleep deprivation disrupts this orderly process, leading to lapses in memory, difficulty concentrating, and impaired decision-making. Over time, these effects can accumulate, setting the stage for more serious cognitive issues. For instance, studies have shown that insufficient sleep in midlife is associated with an increased risk of dementia in later years. The mechanisms behind this link are complex but involve the brain's inability to clear out toxic waste products, such as beta-amyloid proteins, that accumulate during wakefulness.

Emotional regulation is another critical domain influenced by sleep. When we're well-rested, the amygdala, a part of the brain involved in processing emotions, operates in harmony with the prefrontal cortex, the brain's rational decision-maker. But after a night of poor sleep, this balance is disrupted, leaving the amygdala more reactive and the prefrontal cortex less capable of reigning it in. This imbalance can make us more prone to mood swings, heightened stress responses, and even long-term mental health conditions like anxiety and depression.

Interestingly, sleep also influences how old we *feel* — our subjective age. Poor sleep quality can make individuals feel significantly older than they are, not just in perception but in tangible declines in cognitive and emotional health. Conversely, consistent, restorative sleep fosters a sense of vitality and youthfulness.

Keep in mind that the impact of sleep on mental health isn't limited to day-to-day functioning. Over the long term, consistent sleep deprivation is linked to structural changes in the brain, such as reduced gray matter volume in areas crucial for memory and decision-making. That is to say, lack of sleep doesn't just do a number on neurochemicals and hormones, it can actually change the physical architecture of your brain. Yikes.

～⁹

## More Sleep, or More Regular Sleep?

In recent years, a shift in sleep research has illuminated the profound importance of regularity in sleep patterns. It's not just about how much you sleep but also when you sleep, a concept that has upended traditional thinking around rest and health. We now know that irregular sleep patterns —frequently changing bedtimes or wake-up times— can wreak havoc on the body's internal clock, also known as the circadian rhythm. This disruption has a cascading effect on metabolic processes, inflammation regulation, and overall cardiovascular health.

Sleep regularity acts like the steady beat of a drum, maintaining rhythm in the body's complex biological orchestra. When this rhythm is thrown off, the instruments start playing out of sync, creating chaos that impacts every system. People who stick to a consistent sleep schedule have a much lower risk of major health issues. Maintaining regular sleep patterns is associated with up to a 48% lower risk of dying from any cause, a 39% lower risk of dying from cancer, and a 57% lower risk of dying from heart-related conditions compared to those with irregular sleep schedules. It turns out that sleep regularity is an even stronger predictor of long-term health and survival than the total number of hours slept — good news for those of us who might find it difficult to fit in those extra few hours.

Despite its unparalleled benefits, sleep remains undervalued in modern society, often sacrificed at the altar of productivity. Yet the science is clear: sleep is not a passive state of inactivity but an active, restorative process critical for well-being. So if there is one lesson I want you to take away from this chapter, it is that acting to improve both the quality and consistency of your sleep could be one of the most impactful steps you take toward living longer, healthier lives.

# CHAPTER 20

# The Weight of the World: Stress and Aging

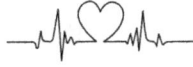

We all know at least one person who happens to look much younger than they actually are. On the flip side, most of us also know at least one person who received the short end of the stick: they look noticeably *older* than their age. If you asked the two about their lives, I would be willing to bet that the older-looking individual has lived a more stressful life. Few things age you like stress — just take a look at any U.S. president before and after their tenure in the oval office.

While it is an unavoidable part of life, the effects of stress linger on long after the fleeting frustrations we might feel in a traffic jam or during a hectic day at work. It doesn't just erode our mental health, it infiltrates the machinery of our cells, accelerating biological aging through mechanisms that are as fascinating as they are concerning.

## A "Cell's-Eye View" of Stress

Stress is often described as the body's fight-or-flight response — a burst of energy meant to help us tackle immediate threats. But when that response is perpetually activated, it starts to wear down our internal systems.

At the cellular level, stress wields its influence by shortening telomeres — remember, these are the protective caps at the ends of our chromosomes. Each time a cell divides, the caps naturally shorten. However, chronic stress speeds up this process, often through elevated levels of cortisol and other stress hormones, which inhibit the enzyme telomerase. Telomerase usually repairs and elongates telomeres, but under stress, its activity diminishes, leaving our DNA vulnerable to damage and decay. Individuals under prolonged stress, such as caregivers or those exposed to early life adversities, often exhibit telomeres resembling those of much older individuals.

The story doesn't stop at telomeres. Chronic stress also disrupts mitochondrial function, a cornerstone of cellular health. Mitochondria produce energy, yes, but they also generate reactive oxygen species as byproducts. These molecules can damage cellular components like DNA, proteins, and lipids if not properly managed. Under normal circumstances, the cell keeps things in balance through its antioxidant defenses — a complex system of enzymes that bind to, and neutralize, the harmful molecules. But stress tilts the scales, amplifying the production of reactive oxygen species and causing damage to mitochondrial DNA. This is more vulnerable to harm than nuclear DNA due to its proximity to the site of production and limited repair mechanisms. Soon, we're facing a downward spiral: damaged mitochondria produce an excess of reactive oxygen species, which in turn further accelerate cellular aging and increase inflammation.

Inflammation is another critical player in the stress-aging nexus. Chronic stress triggers the release of pro-inflammatory cytokines, which can overwhelm the body's ability to regulate immune responses. This inflammaging links stress to age-related diseases like cardiovascular disease, diabetes, and neurodegenerative disorders. Stress-induced inflammation not only damages tissues but also fosters cellular senescence — a state where cells stop dividing but don't die, releasing toxic signals that harm neighboring cells and perpetuate a cycle of aging.

~

## Stress and the Brain: A Vulnerable Organ

Stress is one of the most potent forces shaping the human brain, acting as both a sculptor and a destroyer, depending on its intensity and duration. While short-term stress can enhance alertness and reaction time, chronic stress takes a toll on the brain's structure and function, especially in areas responsible for memory, emotion, and decision-making.

The brain's limbic system, which includes the hippocampus, amygdala, and prefrontal cortex, is especially vulnerable. Chronic exposure to stress hormones like cortisol can shrink the hippocampus, a critical region for memory and learning. The amygdala, responsible for processing emotions, often becomes hyperactive, heightening fear responses and making it harder to regulate emotions. At the same time, the prefrontal cortex, which governs decision-making and impulse control, shows reduced activity and connectivity. This imbalance between the emotional and rational parts of the brain can lead to a vicious cycle: heightened emotional reactivity makes it harder to cope with stress, which in turn makes you more susceptible to stress.

Stress also rewires the brain at the microscopic level. Neural connections weaken, and new growth slows, a process linked to impaired cognitive functions like memory and focus. A recent UK Biobank study highlights how childhood stress, such as abuse or neglect, can leave lasting imprints on the brain's architecture, reducing grey matter in areas like the hippocampus and white matter integrity in pathways that connect critical brain regions. Grey matter consists of the densely packed neurons responsible for processing information and executing tasks, while white matter comprises the communication highways, allowing signals to travel between different brain regions. These changes can persist for decades, increasing the risk of mental health issues like depression and anxiety.

Moreover, chronic stress is a significant driver of neuroinflammation. When stress hormones flood the brain, they activate immune cells called microglia. These cells, meant to protect the brain, can overreact, releasing inflammatory molecules that damage neurons and disrupt brain function. This inflammation is increasingly linked to neurodegenerative diseases like Alzheimer's, where the brain's ability to clear harmful proteins is compromised.

What's really frightening is stress's ability to disrupt the brain's repair mechanisms. Neurogenesis, the process by which the brain generates new neurons, particularly in the hippocampus, is significantly stunted under chronic stress. Without this renewal, the brain struggles to adapt, learn, and recover from injuries.

Yet, the effects of stress aren't uniform. Gender, life stage, and genetics all play a role in determining how stress impacts the brain. For instance, the same UK Biobank study found that women are more likely to experience changes in brain structure due to childhood stress, while men are more affected by stress in adulthood. This gender disparity may stem from differences in hormonal responses to stress and brain development patterns.

Understanding these mechanisms offers a path forward. Strategies like mindfulness, exercise, and social support can buffer the brain against stress, promoting resilience and preserving cognitive function.

~~~

## A Glimpse of Hope? Reversing Stress-Induced Aging

Despite its pervasive effects, stress-induced aging isn't necessarily a one-way street. The biological changes triggered by stress can, in some cases, be reversed. This brings a glimmer of optimism to the complex interplay between stress and aging, showcasing the body's remarkable capacity for resilience and repair.

Stress-induced biological aging is often measured using "epigenetic clocks," tools that assess DNA methylation — chemical modifications to DNA that regulate gene activity (much more on this to come). These clocks have revealed that stressful events like surgery, severe illness, or even pregnancy can temporarily accelerate biological aging.

However, when the stressor is removed, the body begins to heal. A study using mice demonstrated this vividly: young mice surgically paired with older ones, sharing the older animals' blood, showed an increase in biological age. Yet once separated, their biological age returned to baseline, emphasizing the dynamic nature of aging. A similar pattern emerges in humans. For example, individuals recovering from major stressors, such as emergency surgery or severe COVID-19, experienced a temporary spike in biological age that subsided with recovery. This fluctuation suggests that while stress accelerates biological aging, the body retains an intrinsic ability to rebound. Interestingly, certain interventions may enhance this recovery process. For instance, patients treated with the anti-inflammatory drug tocilizumab during severe COVID-19 showed greater reversals in biological age compared to untreated patients, highlighting potential therapeutic pathways for mitigating stress-induced damage.

The mechanisms are deeply rooted in cellular processes. Stress often disrupts homeostasis, the balance essential for cellular function, by elevating levels of reactive oxygen species, inflammatory markers, and other damaging compounds. But when stress subsides, the body's repair systems spring into action. Antioxidants neutralize reactive oxygen species, and epigenetic markers — such as DNA methylation patterns — begin to reset. This ability to "rewind the clock" isn't unlimited but demonstrates that biological age is malleable and influenced by external conditions .

## Managing Stress for Healthy Aging

Understanding the mechanisms by which stress accelerates aging is only half the battle; the real challenge lies in implementing strategies to manage it. Lifestyle factors, like the ones we have been discussing, can play a critical role in recovery. Practices including regular exercise, mindfulness, and restorative sleep have been shown to promote resilience against stress-induced damage. Mindfulness practices, for instance, can reduce cortisol levels, minimizing the long-term impact of stress. Social support and time in nature have also been shown to significantly reduce stress levels and their biological consequences. Meanwhile, cutting-edge research into stress biology is exploring potential pharmaceutical interventions that could target stress-related aging at the molecular level.

In the end, stress is an inevitable part of life, but its impact on aging is far from predetermined. By recognizing its profound effects and taking proactive steps to manage it, we can not only protect our health but also add quality years to our lives.

# CHAPTER 21

# The Power of Connection: Community, Social Bonds, and Longevity

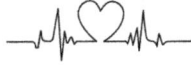

There's a pandemic underway. No, it has nothing to do with viruses or bacteria, or any other pathogen, for that matter. This is a silent pandemic — the pandemic of loneliness. The health consequences, however, are just as serious: social isolation has a bigger impact on mortality than smoking 15 cigarettes a day or having six alcoholic drinks a day.

The alarm bells are finally starting to ring. In 2018, the United Kingdom published the world's first government strategy dedicated to tackling loneliness. Japan followed suit in 2021, appointing a "Minister of Loneliness" to help tackle the issue. Since then, the US has joined the ranks of countries making loneliness an official talking point for policy. And finally, towards the tail-end of 2023, the World Health Organization (WHO) launched a commission to combat global social isolation —a paucity of social connections— and loneliness —the subjective experience of lacking meaningful relationships.

So, what do we know about this silent pandemic, and what can we do about it?

## Older Adults Are Especially Lonely

One of the key findings of research on loneliness is that elderly populations are especially vulnerable to feeling neglected and alone. Indeed, the experience of loneliness across the lifespan tends to follow a U-shaped curve; it is high during our adolescent years as we grapple with life transitions and questions of identity, it lessens somewhat during middle adulthood when we begin to establish families and solidify social networks (whether this be at work or through contact with other parents), and then it increases again sharply once we move into old age.

While this vertiginous uptick in loneliness with age has a variety of causes, one stands out as a prime culprit: a decline in mobility. The older we grow, the more difficult it becomes to perform routine, everyday tasks like walking up stairs or carrying groceries. Often, these activities end up being cut out wholesale, leaving elderly individuals in a state of physical inactivity that jeopardizes their ability to meet and connect with others. They become "prisoners" in their own bodies.

Hearing loss is another major issue. Language is a gateway to community; more often than not, we get to know one another through conversation. Speaking helps bridge gaps and create bonds. But if a person's hearing is compromised, one side of the equation breaks down: conversation is as much about listening as it is about talking. Difficulty hearing creates a barrier in communication, risking a steady decline into loneliness. This is reflected by research on the topic, which suggests that loss of hearing increases the risk of social isolation by up to 28%. And this is not an abstract concern: up to two-thirds of older adults experience hearing loss, yet only around 10 to 30% use hearing aids.

Despite the extent of the loneliness epidemic varying from country to country, the U-shaped trajectory represents a global trend. Whether it be in the U.K., Germany, or Australia, most people begin to feel increasingly lonely as they get older. But some groups, it should be pointed out, are at a higher risk of loneliness than others, including women, those with less education, and those with a lower income.

~~

## Middle-Aged Adults Are Not Immune

Although loneliness is highest in the elderly, it is becoming more of an issue in middle-aged adults as well — the usual U-shaped trajectory may not hold up much longer. Recent research suggests that this is particularly true for middle-aged Americans, who are consistently lonelier than their European counterparts.

By following 53,000 middle-aged adults from the U.S. and 13 European countries for a total of 18 years, the researchers were able to conclude that Americans rank highest when it comes to feelings of social isolation. Those in Mediterranean Europe and England were not far behind, whereas middle-aged adults in Continental and Nordic Europe —think Germany, Sweden, Norway, and so on— reported the lowest levels of loneliness.

Exactly why Americans are more prone to loneliness was not addressed by the study, but the authors venture a guess: "We think that the loneliness Americans are reporting compared to peer nations comes down to limited social safety nets and to cultural norms that prioritize individualism over community." Social isolation is closely linked to poverty, and the U.S. is an expert in poverty; in fact, the U.S. has one of the highest poverty rates of all OECD countries.

Another plausible explanation is America's car-centric culture, which casts aside public space and parks in favor of endless parking lots, behemoth expressways, and suburban developments. In a press release for a study on walkable neighborhoods, James F. Sallis, Ph.D., Distinguished Professor at the Herbert Wertheim School of Public Health, mentions: "Transportation and land-use policies across the U.S. have strongly prioritized car travel and suburban development, so millions of Americans live in neighborhoods where they must drive everywhere, usually alone, and have little or no chance to interact with their neighbors."

The built environment we live in shapes our interactions. When that environment caters predominantly to car travel, we end up with unwalkable cities and a paucity of public space, both of which hinder the possibilities for social interaction and the development of deep community bonds.

## How Harmful Is Loneliness Really?

Alright, so loneliness is on the rise across age groups. That isn't great, but how worried do we really need to be? Beyond the mental health issues that accompany protracted spells of social isolation, there are also a host of risks to physical well-being.

For one, socially isolated people are at a 25% increased risk of cancer-related mortality and a 32% increased risk of strokes. The risk of heart disease also goes up by a staggering 29%. And as far as dementia is concerned, those who are socially isolated are one and a half times more likely to develop issues than people who report having a rich social life.

Another study found that, in patients with heart failure, those who self-described as feeling very lonely were at a three-fold greater risk of death than their non-lonely counterparts. They were also at a 68% increased risk of being hospitalized over the span of a year.

Clearly, loneliness and social isolation are very tightly linked to poor health outcomes. But as always, trying to separate causation from correlation is a messy business; it is not entirely obvious whether we can say loneliness is causing these health issues. It may be that people with certain health issues or disabilities are more prone to loneliness in the first place, in which case the two simply overlap. Still, it is undeniable that social isolation comes hand-in-hand with an increased risk of mortality. Even if it cannot be said to be causing health issues, it is a flare in the night sky warning us that someone is in dire need of help. We need to start paying attention.

~~~

## Expanding Our Vocabulary to Include 'Social Health'

Experts talk at length about the importance of physical health: we need to exercise and follow healthy diets, otherwise we risk running into chronic illnesses like cancer or heart disease. The concept of mental health has also been normalized, and with it, therapy and other preventative approaches. Now, it is time to work another dimension of health into our vernacular: "social health."

What is social health, and why should we care about it? Essentially, it's a metric to gauge someone's well-being along social lines. In the same way we use "physical health" to keep tabs on how we are doing physically, "social health" refers to how we are doing socially; it is about the quantity and quality of human relationships in our lives and whether the deep-rooted need for human connection is being met.

A recent study offers an intuitive way of grasping the idea. The authors introduce their work by sharing a snippet of text by William James, a psychologist active in the late 1800s:

"No more fiendish punishment could be devised, were such a thing physically possible, than that one should be turned loose in society and remain absolutely unnoticed by all the members thereof. If no one turned round when we entered, answered when we spoke, or minded what we did, but if every person we met 'cut us dead', and acted as if we were non-existing things, a kind of rage and impotent despair would ere long well up in us, from which the cruelest bodily tortures would be a relief; for these would make us feel that, however bad might be our plight, we had not sunk to such a depth as to be unworthy of attention at all."

The above scenario is the most extreme example of poor social health: no one even recognizes your existence. There are no relationships to speak of, let alone any meaningful ones. It is not by accident that solitary confinement is considered one of the severest forms of punishment — we all understand, implicitly or otherwise, that human connection is a critical need. And being deprived of this need has serious negative consequences.

Strong social health, on the other hand, is characterized by a sense of being seen and heard, by having a community you are integrated into and can rely on.

Importantly, and not unlike physical or mental health, social health exists along a spectrum and can change over time. Moving to a new city, for example, might be accompanied by a drop in social health while you build up new relationships and connections. The addition of a new park in your neighborhood, on the other hand, may boost social health, even if you already have plenty of fulfilling friendships.

~❧

## Strategies for Boosting Social Health

In an increasingly disconnected world, loneliness and social isolation have emerged as pressing public health concerns. Governments, health organizations, and urban planners are exploring various strategies to tackle this issue, recognizing the profound impact it can have on mental and physical well-being.

One promising approach lies in strengthening social infrastructure through investments in public spaces like parks, libraries, and community centers. These shared spaces facilitate social interaction and connection, providing opportunities for people to gather, engage in activities, and forge meaningful relationships. Additionally, implementing school-based programs that teach healthy relationship skills and designing workplaces that promote social connections can help cultivate a culture of connection from an early age.

Research has shed light on the effectiveness of different intervention strategies, with group interventions, animal therapy, and technology-based interventions showing particular promise. Group sessions foster active participation and interaction, while animal therapy has proven remarkably effective in reducing loneliness, especially in long-term care settings. Technological interventions, such as videoconferencing, have also helped maintain social connections, particularly for older adults.

The very design of our cities can also play a significant role in mitigating or exacerbating loneliness and social isolation. Walkable neighborhoods, access to public transportation, and proximity to green spaces have all been linked to reduced feelings of loneliness. These features encourage people to spend time outdoors, interact with others, and participate in social activities, fostering a sense of community and belonging. Conversely, poorly designed urban environments, characterized by high density, lack of communal spaces, and inadequate maintenance, can contribute to feelings of isolation and disconnection.

~❧

## A Lifeline for Longevity

We need social interaction in the same way we need to eat, and just as hunger is a signal that we are missing something, loneliness is too. It's our brains' way of telling us that there's a deep need that is not being met. In fact, the two even activate the same regions of the brain — when we are lonely, we are being "starved" of meaningful contact. Increasingly, however, the need for contact is being unmet. And the risks that come with prolonged social isolation are starting to show. We are in the middle of another pandemic, only this one is borne out in silence.

As with any health crisis, the first step is acknowledging what is happening. Until we admit that this is an urgent topic in need of attention, nothing will change. The second step is recognizing that this is a systemic problem, meaning that any long-term solutions will also need to address policy, not just individual intervention. When London eliminated cholera in the late 1800s, it was thanks to changes to waste management, not because of a new pharmaceutical. If we are to overcome the loneliness pandemic, we need a similar approach. After all, public health issues are social issues, and vice versa.

# CHAPTER 22

# Not So Fast! A Look at Social Determinants of Health

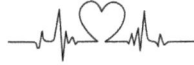

—ₙₗₙ♡₂ₙₗₙ—

It would be remiss of me to talk about the lifestyle decisions that influence our aging journeys without acknowledging that not all of us are in the same position. Sure, eating healthier and exercising more often both sound wonderful, but what if they are decisions that simply aren't available to you? You might recognize that they would improve your longevity prospects —and quality of life— and even *want* to do more of both, yet not be able to regardless. Why? Well, unfortunately, we do not live in an equal society. Certain things, including many of the aforementioned lifestyle choices, lie behind a "paywall" — if you don't have the resources, they remain beyond your grasp.

This brings up a crucial concession: the *desire* to make healthier choices is often not the main determinant of whether you can *actualize* those choices. Lifestyle "choices" aren't always personal choices (and we veer into dangerous territory when we conflate the two). Instead, we have to recognize that they are shaped and constrained by systemic, socioeconomic factors.

The medical community has a term for these non-medical variables that influence health outcomes, *social determinants of health (SODH)*. Per the World Health Organization, they encompass "the conditions in which people are born, grow, work, live, and age, and the wider set of forces and systems shaping the conditions of daily life. These forces and systems include economic policies and systems, development agendas, social norms, social policies and political systems."

~◦

## Nickel-and-dimed: The Longevity Divide

In America's poorest neighborhoods, a silent crisis unfolds daily, robbing children of years of life before they even take their first breath. The bleak reality is that a child born into poverty faces a staggering 10-year reduction in lifespan compared to their affluent counterparts. This gap between rich and poor is not just a statistic; it's a chasm that swallows dreams, potential, and human lives.

The tragedy deepens when we consider how this divide has evolved. From 2001 to 2014, while the wealthiest Americans celebrated an increase of approximately three years in their life expectancy, the poorest saw no improvement. And the gulf keeps widening: whereas the longevity gap stood at 12.6 years in 2000, it increased to a staggering 20.4 years in 2021. This is a damning indictment of a system that allows the rich to thrive while the poor struggle to survive.

It's a sad reminder of how profoundly one's zip code can determine one's fate. Individuals in affluent neighborhoods benefit from cleaner environments, safer streets, and better schools — all factors that contribute to overall health. Conversely, those in low-income areas often experience "neighborhood effects" that negatively impact their health. These include higher crime rates, limited green spaces for physical activity, and inadequate public services.

For example, in New York City, residents of wealthy Upper East Side neighborhoods can expect to live nearly a decade longer than those in the Bronx. This disparity underscores how geographic and economic privilege are inextricably linked. Urban planning and policy decisions often prioritize affluent areas, further entrenching these divides.

~

## The More You Know, The Older You Grow? Education as Longevity Boost

The classroom, often seen as a gateway to opportunity, is also a silent ally in the battle for longevity. With each additional year of education, the risk of premature death diminishes, revealing the profound interplay between learning and life expectancy. Education, as it turns out, is not just a pathway to a better job or social mobility — it is also a cornerstone of public health.

~

## Unequal Opportunities, Unequal Outcomes

Imagine two children born in the same hospital on the same day. Over the decades, their lives diverge, not only due to luck or genetics but due to the number of years spent in school. Research underscores this reality, showing that each additional year of schooling reduces the risk of mortality by 2%. For those who achieve a college degree, their risk of dying early plummets by over 34%, an effect comparable to the life-extending benefits of eating a balanced diet or maintaining a regular exercise regimen.

But how does education translate into longer lives? Education equips individuals with critical thinking skills and health literacy, empowering them to make informed decisions about diet, exercise, and preventive care. It also opens doors to stable employment with health benefits, reducing stress and providing access to resources that support healthy living. Conversely, those with limited education often find themselves in low-wage, high-stress jobs, where exposure to occupational hazards and lack of healthcare exacerbate health risks.

While the connection between education and health is well-documented, access to quality education remains deeply inequitable. Take, for example, the profound differences between a well-resourced suburban school and an underfunded urban counterpart. In one, students benefit from small class sizes, experienced teachers, and college preparatory programs. In the other, classrooms are overcrowded, teachers are underpaid and overstretched, and students often face the added burden of food insecurity or housing instability. This divergence sets the stage for vastly different health and life outcomes.

~♪

## Education as a Shield Against Stress and Disease

Education also acts as a buffer against the chronic stressors that wear down the body over time. Research shows that individuals with higher levels of education are better equipped to navigate life's challenges, using adaptive coping mechanisms that mitigate stress and its physiological effects. Chronic stress, which is more prevalent among those with limited education, contributes to inflammation, cardiovascular disease, and accelerated aging at the cellular level.

The disparities extend to mental health. Studies reveal that higher education correlates with lower rates of depression and anxiety, likely because of increased access to social support networks and mental health services. In contrast, those with less education are more likely to experience social isolation and stigma, compounding their mental health challenges.

~~●

## Programs That Make a Difference

Innovative programs are addressing these disparities, offering hope and measurable success. In Chicago, the Becoming A Man (BAM) initiative has made significant strides in keeping at-risk youth engaged in school. By providing mentoring and cognitive behavioral therapy, BAM not only improves academic performance but also reduces violent crime arrests by 50%, creating a safer and healthier environment for these students to thrive.

On a broader scale, policies like Healthy School Meals for All aim to reduce food insecurity among students, ensuring that every child has the nutrition needed to focus and succeed academically. Such programs recognize that education and health are deeply intertwined, with each reinforcing the other in an upward spiral.

Education is more than a social good; it is a matter of life and death. By ensuring equitable access to quality education, we can unlock the potential for longer, healthier lives for all. The question is not whether we can afford to invest in education — it's whether we can afford not to.

~~9

## "Food Deserts": When There's No Healthy Option

In a country as prosperous as the United States, the existence of food deserts —areas where fresh, nutritious food is scarce —seems almost paradoxical. Yet for millions of Americans, the challenge of accessing affordable, healthy food is a daily reality. These barren zones, where convenience stores and fast-food outlets vastly outnumber grocery stores, are more than an inconvenience, they're a public health crisis. Food deserts reveal the deeper inequities woven into the fabric of society, where your zip code can dictate not just what you eat but how long you live.

~~9

## A Legacy of Redlining and Structural Inequality

To understand the roots of food deserts, we must look to history. Decades of discriminatory policies, such as redlining, have shaped the landscapes of modern cities. In the 1930s, federal agencies marked certain neighborhoods — often home to minority communities — as "hazardous" for investment. Banks refused to lend, businesses moved elsewhere, and these neighborhoods were left to languish. Over time, grocery stores and other essential services disappeared, leaving behind food deserts where fresh produce is a rarity and fast food reigns supreme.

The scars of these policies are still visible today. A 2022 study found that neighborhoods once redlined are significantly more likely to lack access to grocery stores. These areas also tend to face higher rates of poverty, unemployment, and poor health outcomes. The intersection of race and income is unmistakable; predominantly Black and Hispanic neighborhoods are disproportionately affected, underscoring how systemic racism continues to shape access to basic necessities like food.

~●

## The Health Toll of Food Deserts

Imagine a neighborhood where the nearest fresh apple is miles away, but greasy fast food beckons from every corner. This is the daily reality for millions of Americans trapped in food deserts. In New York City alone, an estimated 750,000 residents live in these nutritional wastelands, predominantly in Black and Hispanic neighborhoods like Bedford-Stuyvesant, Brownsville, the South Bronx, and parts of Harlem.

The irony is palpable: in one of the world's wealthiest cities, entire communities struggle to access the essential elements of a healthy diet. It's a cruel twist of fate that in these food deserts, the most readily available sustenance often comes from highly processed, sugar-laden products that contribute to these communities' health problems.

Without full-service supermarkets, residents of food deserts often turn to corner stores, bodegas, and fast-food outlets. These establishments, while convenient, rarely stock fresh produce or other nutritious options. Instead, their shelves are lined with chips, sugary drinks, and other processed foods with little nutritional value but plenty of empty calories.

LaToya Meaders, in an interview with PIXII, paints a vivid picture: "There isn't like a fresh salad in these communities. Think about when you go into a corner bodega. Think about the options inside that store — potato chips, high fructose corn syrup drinks, and everything that is not good for the body."

While these options may be cheaper upfront, they come with a hidden cost: increased rates of obesity, diabetes, heart disease, and even certain cancers. It's no coincidence that communities with the highest concentrations of food deserts often report some of the worst health outcomes in the country. In Chicago, a study found that the death rate from diabetes in food deserts was twice that of areas with access to grocery stores. In California, adults over 50 from Black and brown communities had double the diabetes rate of their white counterparts. These statistics are not just numbers; they represent lives cut short, families torn apart, and communities trapped in a cycle of poor health and diminished opportunity.

For children growing up in these areas, the consequences are particularly dire. Poor nutrition during critical developmental years can lead to long-term cognitive and physical impairments. Schools in food desert regions often report higher rates of absenteeism, lower academic performance, and increased behavioral issues. It's a vicious cycle where limited food access perpetuates poverty and poor health, robbing communities of their potential.

~~

## The Road Ahead: Solutions to Food Insecurity

Addressing food deserts requires more than just opening a few grocery stores. It demands systemic changes to the way we think about food access, urban planning, and community investment. One promising initiative is the Healthy Food Financing Initiative, which has helped fund nearly 1,000 new food retailers in underserved areas. However, as successful as these programs are, they are only part of the solution.

Transportation is another critical piece of the puzzle. For many families living in food deserts, the nearest grocery store might be several miles away, with no reliable public transportation to get there. Expanding transit options or creating mobile grocery stores that bring fresh food directly to neighborhoods can help bridge this gap.

Additionally, urban agriculture offers a way for communities to reclaim agency over their food supply. Community gardens, rooftop farms, and hydroponic systems not only provide fresh produce but also foster a sense of ownership and pride within neighborhoods. These initiatives can help combat the alienation and disempowerment that often accompany life in a food desert.

## Food Deserts and the Fight for Equity

Ultimately, the issue of food deserts is not just about nutrition; it's about equity. The fact that millions of Americans lack access to something as fundamental as healthy food is a salient reminder of the disparities that persist in our society. Tackling this problem will require more than policy changes; it will demand a cultural shift in how we value community health and well-being.

## Toxic Air, Toxic Water, Toxic Health

In 2014, officials in the city of Flint, Michigan switched the water supply to the corrosive Flint River to save money — the consequences were catastrophic. Lead from aging pipes leached into the drinking water, exposing thousands of residents, including an estimated 9,000 children, to neurotoxic levels of the heavy metal. The fallout was swift and devastating: a surge in developmental delays among children, an outbreak of Legionnaires' disease, and widespread mistrust in government institutions. Flint became a symbol of environmental injustice, where decisions driven by economic constraints and political neglect disproportionately harmed an already vulnerable community.

But Flint's story is not an isolated one. Across the United States, low-income and minority communities are routinely subjected to environmental hazards, from polluted air to contaminated water. These inequities are not merely accidental; they are rooted in decades of discriminatory policies like redlining and industrial zoning that have concentrated environmental risks in marginalized areas.

~❧

## Air Pollution: A Silent Predator

Imagine growing up in a neighborhood where the air itself is a threat. In Houston's Manchester district, for example, the air carries a cocktail of toxic chemicals emitted by nearby refineries and chemical plants. Benzene, a known carcinogen, is a constant presence, and children in Manchester are 56% more likely to get leukemia than those living in different parts of Houston.

Across the country, air pollution is responsible for an estimated 200,000 premature deaths annually, with communities of color and low-income neighborhoods bearing the brunt of this burden.

How does polluted air accelerate aging and erode health? The answer lies in its ability to cause oxidative stress and inflammation. Particulate matter (PM2.5), one of the most harmful air pollutants, is small enough to penetrate deep into the lungs and even enter the bloodstream. Once inside, it triggers the production of reactive oxygen species, which damage cells, proteins, and DNA. Over time, this leads to chronic inflammation, a key driver of diseases like asthma, cardiovascular disease, and cancer.

Research has also revealed the epigenetic effects of air pollution. For example, exposure to PM2.5 can alter DNA methylation patterns, effectively switching genes on or off in ways that predispose individuals to chronic illnesses. A 2021 study found that these changes can amplify the risk of respiratory and cardiovascular conditions, disproportionately affecting communities situated near highways and industrial zones.

But beyond the immediate health impacts, there are long-term consequences for education, economic opportunity, and social mobility. Children growing up in polluted environments are more likely to miss school due to illness, struggle with cognitive development, and face lifelong health challenges that limit their potential.

## The Climate Factor: Heat and Flooding

Environmental injustices are magnified by climate change, which acts as a force multiplier for existing disparities. Take heat waves, for example. In Chicago's deadly 1995 heat wave, over 700 lives were lost, predominantly in low-income, predominantly Black neighborhoods. These areas lacked the green spaces and air conditioning that could have mitigated the impact of extreme heat. Urban heat islands — areas where temperatures are significantly higher due to dense infrastructure and sparse vegetation — are more common in disadvantaged neighborhoods, exacerbating health risks during heat waves.

Flooding is another facet of this crisis. As sea levels rise and extreme weather events become more frequent, low-income communities often find themselves on the front lines. The Lower Ninth Ward in New Orleans, a predominantly Black neighborhood, was devastated by Hurricane Katrina and remains vulnerable to future storms. These areas are frequently located in floodplains or low-lying regions, a legacy of discriminatory housing policies that restricted access to safer, more desirable locations.

~ゝ

## Water Pollution: Beyond Flint

Flint may have captured headlines, but water contamination is a widespread issue. In rural communities across the Midwest, agricultural runoff laden with nitrates seeps into groundwater, contaminating drinking supplies. Nitrates, which can interfere with the blood's ability to carry oxygen, are particularly dangerous for infants, increasing the risk of "blue baby syndrome." Meanwhile, in urban areas, aging infrastructure leads to the leaching of heavy metals like lead into drinking water.

The health impacts of contaminated water extend beyond immediate poisoning. Chronic exposure to pollutants like lead has been linked to developmental delays, hypertension, and kidney damage. In communities already grappling with limited access to healthcare, these effects can trap residents in a cycle of illness and economic hardship.

~♪

## The Path Forward: Toward Environmental Justice

Addressing environmental inequities requires more than technical fixes; it demands systemic change. Initiatives like Los Angeles' Clean Up Green Up program, which imposes stricter regulations on industrial polluters in low-income neighborhoods, offer a glimpse of what is possible. Similarly, green infrastructure projects like New York City's Cool Neighborhoods program, which increases urban greenery to combat heat islands, highlight the potential for innovative solutions.

Yet, these efforts are just the beginning. To achieve true environmental justice, policymakers must prioritize the health and well-being of vulnerable communities in all aspects of urban planning and environmental regulation. This includes stricter enforcement of pollution controls, equitable climate adaptation strategies, and robust investments in green spaces for underserved areas.

As we confront the twin challenges of environmental degradation and climate change, we must recognize that their impacts are unequal. At its core, the fight for clean air, safe neighborhoods, and climate resilience is a fight for social justice. It's a battle we cannot afford to lose for the sake of those who have already endured too much and for the generations yet to come.

# PART III

# What Can *Medicine* Do?

# CHAPTER 23

# Reading the Body's Signals: Biomarkers of Aging and Mortality

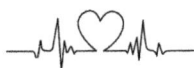

—᠕᠊᠊᠊᠊᠊᠊᠊᠊᠊᠊᠊᠊᠊᠊

A ging is one of life's universal constants, yet it unfolds at dramatically different rates for each individual. While we all count our chronological age in years, the true story of aging lies beneath the surface, in the biological processes that dictate our functional decline. This difference between chronological age — the number of candles on your birthday cake — and biological age — the state of your cells and tissues — is at the heart of the search for reliable biomarkers of aging.

Biomarkers are measurable indicators of biological states or conditions, and in the context of aging, they provide a lens through which we can examine the complicated interplay of genetics, environment, and lifestyle that shapes the aging process. They allow us to ask critical questions: How old is this individual, biologically? How well are their systems functioning? And, perhaps most intriguingly, can we slow, halt, or even reverse aspects of aging?

The importance of biomarkers in longevity research cannot be overstated. They serve as our biological dashboards, helping researchers and clinicians monitor the progression of aging at cellular, tissue, and systemic levels. From molecular markers like DNA-methylation patterns and telomere length to physiological metrics like the stiffness of your arteries and the speed of your metabolism, these tools open a window into the unseen world of aging processes.

Beyond their role in diagnosis, biomarkers are helpful in exploring new avenues for the "treatment" of aging. After all, the first step in developing successful interventions is locating appropriate targets — you can't hit an invisible enemy. Once you know where to look, you can begin to plan and strategize.

Of course, once scientists have developed a potential new anti-aging drug, they still need a way to test its effectiveness. Here, again, biomarkers of age come in handy. Without reliable metrics, the effectiveness of cutting-edge therapies — be it dietary changes, pharmaceuticals, or genetic modifications — would remain speculative at best. Biomarkers allow us to measure success, providing tangible evidence of whether an intervention is genuinely extending health span and life span or simply masking the symptoms of aging.

In the grander scheme, biomarkers also redefine how we think about aging itself. They help shift the narrative from one of inevitability to one of intervention, suggesting that aging is not merely a passive march toward decline but a dynamic process that can be studied, quantified, and potentially altered. As we move deeper into the era of precision medicine, the ability to tailor interventions based on an individual's unique biological age offers a tantalizing glimpse into a future where aging is not just a condition to be managed, but a challenge to be overcome.

## Epigenetic Clocks: Measuring Time in the Body

Every person has their own particular genome, or the entire set of DNA found in their cells. This DNA is fixed, handed down to them by their parents. But although a person's DNA sequence itself won't change over the course of their life, the way in which it is *expressed* will. This is called epigenetics. Essentially, changes that happen "on top of" your DNA that affect the way your genes operate. These modifications serve as a powerful regulatory mechanism, akin to sticky notes placed on a manuscript to signal which chapters to read and which to skip. Epigenetic changes are spurred on by behavioral and environmental factors, including diet, exercise, exposure to pollution, and so on.

One of the central mechanisms of epigenetic change is called DNA methylation, which happens when chemical methyl groups are added to DNA. By attaching themselves to a section of DNA, these methyl groups act like "on" or "off" switches, governing whether genes in that section are expressed. Since these changes don't impact the DNA sequence itself, they are technically reversible. But why does this happen? The prevailing theory is that methylation changes are part of an organism's attempt to manage gene expression dynamically, adapting to the challenges of time and wear.

From these changes in DNA methylation arose a groundbreaking innovation: *epigenetic clocks*. The first of these was developed by Steve Horvath, a biostatistician whose early fascination with aging and longevity began in high school. As a teenager in Germany, Horvath, his twin brother, and a friend formed what they called "The Gilgamesh Project," inspired by the ancient Sumerian epic about the quest for eternal youth. This youthful curiosity blossomed into a career dedicated to decoding the molecular mechanisms of aging.

The key to understanding epigenetic clocks is the discovery that DNA methylation is correlated with age. The DNA of people of similar chronological age is methylated in similar places. This means there is a predictable pattern to the way our DNA is methylated that can be traced through time. In a sense, the methylation patterns are like numbers on a clock that we have slowly learned to decipher. By understanding these patterns, we can predict a person's age just by looking at a snapshot of their epigenome.

Certain people may have a DNA methylation pattern that runs ahead of their chronological age — their DNA looks "old" for their age. This is called epigenetic age acceleration. And, of course, there are also the lucky ones whose DNA looks "young" for their age.

Horvath's clock was the result of painstaking analysis of DNA methylation data from over 13,000 tissue samples. His mathematical model could estimate an individual's biological age — defined as the functional, rather than chronological, state of their body. This innovation was a leap forward because it allowed researchers to measure aging more precisely than ever before. Unlike other methods, such as telomere length measurement, epigenetic clocks could assess age across multiple tissues with remarkable accuracy.

Horvath's work didn't stop there. His second-generation clock, aptly named GrimAge, incorporated additional markers to predict not just biological age but also morbidity and mortality risks. It's no wonder the epigenetic clock has been dubbed the "gold standard" in the emerging field of biohorology—the science of measuring time in living systems.

~~♪~~

## The Consumer Revolution: Longevity Startups and Personalized Health

Epigenetic clocks are no longer confined to the sterile environments of research labs — they've made their way into the burgeoning world of consumer-focused longevity startups. Companies like Elysium Health and MyDNAge have brought epigenetic age testing directly to consumers, offering saliva or blood-based tests that promise to reveal your "real age." These services, often marketed as cutting-edge wellness products, allow individuals to measure their biological age and track it over time, much like monitoring weight or cholesterol levels.

The appeal of these tests is clear: they provide a quantifiable metric of aging and empower users to make data-driven health decisions. For example, a consumer might adjust their diet, exercise routine, or supplement intake based on the results, then retest months later to see if these changes have slowed their biological clock. This feedback loop creates a sense of agency in a realm that has traditionally felt immutable.

Yet, there's also a risk that the commercial availability of epigenetic clocks oversimplifies complex science. While the tests provide an age estimate, they rarely account for the myriad factors influencing methylation patterns, such as immune cell composition or environmental exposures. A saliva test indicating a "younger" biological age might not reflect the health of critical systems like the cardiovascular or nervous systems, leading to a false sense of security.

Still, the integration of epigenetic clocks into consumer health represents an exciting shift. As technologies improve, these tools could evolve from wellness products into essential components of preventive medicine. Imagine a future where annual health check-ups include a detailed epigenetic report, providing insights into an individual's aging trajectory and early warnings for age-related diseases.

~~●

## Causation or Correlation? The Limits of Epigenetic Clocks

While epigenetic clocks are celebrated for their precision in estimating biological age, they remain the subject of considerable scientific debate. One of the primary criticisms lies in their inability to distinguish between causation and correlation. DNA methylation changes are undoubtedly associated with aging, but are they drivers of the aging process or merely byproducts of it? This distinction is crucial for their utility as both biomarkers and therapeutic targets.

Some researchers argue that methylation patterns captured by epigenetic clocks might reflect an organism's adaptive responses to aging rather than its underlying causes. For instance, "adaptive methylation" could act as a protective mechanism, mitigating the effects of cellular damage. If true, current epigenetic clocks may actually be measuring two independent variables: aging and adaptive responses. It also means that targeting methylation changes to reverse aging might inadvertently disrupt beneficial, adaptive processes.

Luckily, we're making some progress towards addressing this concern. A study released in early 2024 by an international group of researchers —spread across a heavy-hitting list of universities, including Harvard Medical School, Stanford University, UCLA, and the University of Lausanne— pushes beyond the limitations of existing epigenetic clocks by introducing *causality-enriched* models that separate DNA methylation changes into two categories: damage-related (DamAge) and adaptation-related (AdaptAge). By untangling the two, the findings help us get a sense of which methylation sites we might be able to target to reverse aging, and which sites we need to make sure to keep our hands off.

Other critics highlight that the clocks are often trained on large datasets using machine learning, which identifies patterns without necessarily elucidating mechanisms. This black-box approach means that while the clocks are mathematically robust, their biological interpretations are less clear. For example, the GrimAge clock predicts mortality risk with impressive accuracy, but it remains uncertain whether the methylation sites it leverages are directly involved in the processes leading to death.

The reliance on blood samples for most epigenetic clocks also raises questions about their generalizability. Blood is accessible and easy to sample, but it may not accurately represent aging processes in other tissues, such as the brain or liver. The development of tissue-specific clocks could address this limitation but would require significant time and resources.

Despite these challenges, one thing is clear: DNA methylation and epigenetic clocks are reshaping our understanding of aging. Whether as research aids, diagnostic tools, or personal health metrics, the significance of epigenetic clocks as biomarkers is hard to overstate.

~~•

## Omics Research: A New Lens on Aging

Omics research is the science of scale. It refers to a suite of powerful technologies that capture vast amounts of biological data from DNA, RNA, proteins, metabolites, and even the microbiome, allowing scientists to examine the interplay of life's molecular components. When combined, known as "multi-omics," the data allow us to move beyond a single gene or protein and instead take a systems-level approach. This lets us map the networks and pathways that govern aging and disease at the broadest level.

You might think of aging as an orchestra of sorts, where each "instrument" — whether a gene, protein, or metabolite — plays a role in the symphony of life. Over time, the music shifts, with some instruments going out of tune or dropping out altogether. Omics helps us understand these changes in unprecedented detail, providing insights into how biological processes break down over time.

The pioneering of omics research has also enabled a fundamental shift in approach. Usually, science advances through hypothesis testing. That is, researchers come up with an educated guess —a hypothesis— which they use as a starting point for further investigation. They design an experiment around this guess and see whether the evidence supports it or not. Hypothesis first, data second. But with omics research, which can amass huge sums of information at once, scientists can now flip the established process on its head: data first, hypothesis second. Essentially, we can now gather data "blindly" and, with the help of machine learning and other AI technologies, search the data for patterns. Patterns which, it should be noted, we may otherwise never have been able to recognize (or hypothesize). Thus, we enter an era of "hypothesis-free" research.

~~✎

## Genomics: The Blueprint of Life

Genomics represents the foundation of omics research, focusing on the complete set of DNA that defines an organism. This "blueprint of life" contains the instructions for building and maintaining the body, encoded in sequences of adenine (A), cytosine (C), guanine (G), and thymine (T). Each of us carries a unique genomic fingerprint, yet we share over 99% of our DNA with every other human on Earth. It's within the remaining 1% — the genetic variants — that the secrets to aging and longevity are written.

## What Role Does Genomics Play in Aging?

At its core, aging reflects a gradual decline in the body's ability to maintain homeostasis and repair itself. While environmental and lifestyle factors contribute to this decline, genomics offers insight into the biological mechanisms that set the stage for how we age. Genetic variants can determine susceptibility to age-related diseases, influence how our bodies respond to stress, and even impact overall lifespan. For instance, twin studies suggest that up to 30% of the variation in human longevity is heritable, though other research places this figure closer to 16% (and, in some cases, as low as 10%).

In recent years, large-scale genome-wide association studies (GWAS) have become a cornerstone of aging research, helping scientists identify specific genetic loci — regions of the genome — associated with traits such as lifespan, healthspan, and extreme longevity. Genome-wide association studies work by comparing the genomes of thousands — or even hundreds of thousands — of individuals to pinpoint genetic variants that are more common in those who share a particular trait, such as living beyond 90 years or developing age-related diseases. This approach has revealed a treasure trove of insights, linking certain genes to aging mechanisms and offering potential targets for therapeutic interventions. Notable findings include the *FOXO3* gene, which appears to play a role in stress resistance and cellular repair, and the *APOE* gene, which is associated with Alzheimer's and cardiovascular disease.

## FOXO3: The Longevity Gene

Among the pantheon of aging-related genes, *FOXO3* stands out as a particularly intriguing figure. Known as a "longevity gene," variants of *FOXO3* are disproportionately found in centenarians worldwide, from Japan to Germany.

But what exactly does *FOXO3* do to earn its reputation as a longevity gene? When activated, *FOXO3* travels to the nucleus — the command center of the cell — where it orchestrates the expression of genes involved in stress resistance, DNA repair, metabolism, and cellular maintenance.

When it comes to DNA repair, *FOXO3* steps in by activating genes central to DNA repair processes, such as nucleotide excision repair (NER) and homologous recombination. These pathways work to identify and fix errors in the DNA sequence, preserving the cell's genetic integrity and preventing the accumulation of potentially harmful mutations. *FOXO3* also promotes autophagy, which, you'll recall, is vital for maintaining a tidy and efficient cellular environment.

Beyond its role in safeguarding DNA, *FOXO3* is a critical player in managing oxidative stress by boosting the production of antioxidant enzymes. Some of these enzymes convert highly reactive superoxide radicals into less harmful molecules, while others further detoxify these by breaking them down into even smaller, more benign components. Together, such enzymes act like a molecular cleanup crew, reducing the cellular wear and tear caused by oxidative stress.

One of *FOXO3*'s most crucial roles is preserving stem cell populations. Stem cells, remember, are like our body's reserve of "spare parts," vital for tissue regeneration and repair. By maintaining these cellular backups, FOXO3 helps the body retain its ability to heal and regenerate even as it ages.

Of course, the nature of our genome is such that we have no say over it — it's down to the roll of the dice. But while we can't change the *FOXO3* variants we inherit, emerging research suggests we can influence the activity of this longevity gene. Think of *FOXO3* as having a dimmer switch that we can adjust through lifestyle choices.

For example, caloric restriction activates *FOXO3* in a variety of organisms. Similarly, certain types of exercise can increase *FOXO3* expression in human skeletal muscle, boosting its protective effects. Even specific nutrients, like resveratrol (found in red wine), have been shown to enhance *FOXO3* activity through related pathways. This suggests that even if you didn't win the genetic lottery, you still have tools to influence how this gene works in your favor.

I know you're growing tired of all these lifestyle interventions. So, what can *medicine* do? Well, scientists are exploring ways to directly enhance the activity of *FOXO3* using pharmacological and genetic approaches. Small-molecule activators designed to boost the gene-function pharmacologically are already being tested. Gene-therapy approaches that increase *FOXO3* expression in specific tissues could provide targeted benefits, and epigenetic strategies to modulate *FOXO3* activity without altering the genetic code are another promising avenue of research. While much work remains, the pathways governed by *FOXO3* represent exciting targets for interventions aimed at improving healthspan and potentially extending lifespan.

## APOE: A Genetic Puzzle in Longevity and Health

Not all genes associated with longevity offer simple, clear-cut advantages. The *APOE* gene is a prime example of this complexity. Known for its role in cholesterol metabolism, *APOE* functions like a molecular Swiss Army knife, its variants influencing a range of processes critical to our health and longevity. The gene comes in three main forms, or alleles: *E2, E3*, and *E4*. Though these variants differ by just one or two amino acids, their effects on our bodies can be profound.

The *E2* variant is often celebrated as a longevity gene. Frequently found in centenarians, it is associated with a noticeably reduced risk of Alzheimer's disease. This is especially true for people with the good fortune of inheriting two copies of the *APOE E2* variant — every person inherits two copies of each gene —one from each parent— which creates various combinations of genetic variants. Among autopsy-confirmed cases, having two *E2* alleles reduced the risk of Alzheimer's by 66% compared to those with one *E2* and one *E3* allele, by 87% compared to individuals with two *E3* alleles, and by an astounding 99.6% compared to those carrying two *E4* alleles.

What's the secret? How is the *E2* variant protecting us from Alzheimer's disease? Although we are a longshot from having a full understanding of the mechanisms (or of the disease, for that matter), we know a couple of things. For one, the protective power of the *APOE E2* variant appears to hinge on its ability to help the brain manage one of the condition's main culprits: amyloid-β (Aβ). Amyloid-β is a sticky protein that, as it builds up, forms plaques that disrupt communication between brain cells and trigger widespread damage. People with the *E2* variant tend to clear amyloid-β from their brains more efficiently, preventing these harmful plaques from forming. This process involves better support from microglia — the brain's cleanup crew — and more effective transport of amyloid-β out of the brain through the blood-brain barrier, a protective filter that controls what enters and exits the brain.

But *APOE E2*'s benefits go beyond just plaque prevention. It also supports the brain's overall health, reducing inflammation and helping neurons — the cells responsible for thinking and memory — stay strong and connected. In essence, *E2* promotes a calmer, more balanced immune environment. This means less collateral damage and a brain better equipped to handle the challenges of aging.

Aside from Alzheimer's disease, the *E2* variant is known to reduce the risk of cardiovascular issues. This protective effect can be traced to its biochemistry: *E2* binds less effectively to the low-density lipoprotein (LDL) receptor. This leads to a slower clearance of very low-density lipoproteins (VLDL) and results in lower LDL cholesterol levels in the bloodstream. It's as though *E2* provides a natural cholesterol-lowering mechanism, helping to keep arteries clear and supporting overall cardiovascular health.

On the other end of the spectrum lies the so-called "troublemaker," the *E4* variant. Carriers of this allele face an increased risk of both Alzheimer's disease and cardiovascular problems. In the brain, *E4* is less efficient at clearing beta-amyloid and appears to impair the function of the blood-brain barrier, potentially allowing harmful substances to enter the brain more easily. It also alters the activity of microglia, the brain's immune cells, making them more prone to inflammation. And when it comes to the heart, *E4* binds more tightly to the LDL receptor, which leads to faster clearance of very low-density lipoproteins (VLDL) but higher overall LDL cholesterol levels. Not good.

Interestingly, the *APOE* gene's effects are not confined to the brain or cardiovascular system. It also plays a role in immune function. Evidence suggests that *E4* carriers may have altered responses to infections, possibly reflecting an evolutionary adaptation. In environments where parasitic diseases were common, *E4* might have offered a survival advantage, even as it introduced vulnerabilities to diseases more relevant in today's longer-lived populations.

Alright, that's a lot of information — but what does it mean for *you?* Well, understanding your *APOE* status can provide valuable insights for personalized health planning. For those with the *E4* variant, proactive measures to protect cardiovascular and brain health may be essential. This could include regular cholesterol checks, timely interventions with medications if needed, and lifestyle choices that promote brain health, such as consistent exercise. While universally beneficial, these steps may be particularly critical for anyone who is an *E4* carrier and is aiming to mitigate their heightened risks.

## "Actionable Genes": Forewarned is Forearmed

*APOE4* is an extreme example of a "bad luck" gene. Yet, there are a large number of other genes that are linked to significantly reduced lifespan due to their connection with serious diseases. These are the termed "actionable genes," and they come in many flavors.

For instance, pathogenic variants in the *BRCA2* gene can cut life expectancy by up to seven years due to an increased risk of cancers like breast and ovarian cancer. Similarly, mutations in the LDL receptor gene (*LDLR*), which affects cholesterol metabolism, are associated with early-onset cardiovascular disease. Recent studies suggest that carriers of such genes may live anywhere from three to 15 years fewer than their noncarrier counterparts.

But they are called *actionable* for a reason: these are genes that are known to increase the risk of a disease *for which there is a therapeutic intervention.* As such, with the right medical treatment, their negative health effects can be limited or prevented entirely.

The term first gained traction in 2013, after the American College of Medical Genetics and Genomics (ACMG) published guidelines on how to report secondary findings; that is, findings regarding potentially harmful variants of a gene unrelated to the primary objective of testing. Basically, a way of keeping tabs on different versions of genes. Since then, the organization has updated the list of actionable genes regularly. And in 2021, it announced that the list would be updated once a year to help stay on top of newly discovered genetic variants with negative health effects.

Based on large genomic studies, roughly 4% percent of the population in the United Kingdom and in the United States carry actionable genes. Although such genes can absolutely be life-shortening, they needn't be: population-wide genetic screening can help flag individuals who are predisposed to cancer, heart disease, kidney disease, and so on. Armed with this knowledge, patients and healthcare providers can design disease-prevention and treatment programs tailored to the individual. From heart disease to cancer, early detection and intervention are crucial to improving health outcomes.

Unfortunately, while we have the tools for large-scale genetic sequencing —and the need for it— we're lacking political will and policy. Initiatives such as the "All of Us" Research Program, founded in the United States in 2015 during Barack Obama's tenure as president, are a step in the right direction. Still, such programs are currently the exception when they should be the norm. For lack of a better alternative, people frequently turn to at-home testing kits for answers; unfortunately, these are wildly inaccurate. Genetic sequencing needs to become a routine part of medical checkups in early life to help inform patients and devise effective, individualized health programs.

Until then, go out and bother your doctor for a genetic test, it just might grant you another three years of life, or 15.

~ 9

## Transcriptomics: The Gene's Voice

If genomics provides the instructions, transcriptomics captures how those instructions are carried out. At its core, transcriptomics focuses on RNA, the molecular messengers that carry the instructions from DNA to the cellular machinery responsible for making proteins. These RNA molecules offer a snapshot of which genes are "on" or "off" in a given cell at a given moment. This proves an invaluable tool for studying aging, as it provides insight into how gene expression shifts over time and in response to stress, disease, or environmental factors.

## How Transcriptomics Works as a Biomarker of Aging

Aging leaves a distinct mark on the transcriptome — the collection of all RNA molecules in a cell. By deciphering these marks, we can build a sense of how old someone might be just by looking at the RNA in their cells. For instance, genes involved in inflammation often ramp up, contributing to chronic low-grade inflammation. At the same time, genes tied to processes like repair and stress resistance may become less active.

One standout factor is the role of transcript length in aging. RNA transcripts are the molecular messengers that carry instructions from DNA to the machinery in the cell responsible for building proteins. Think of them as an instruction manual used by someone putting together furniture — each transcript tells the cell what to make and how to make it. These transcripts vary in length, depending on the size of the gene they are derived from. Longer transcripts come from larger, more complex genes that often encode proteins essential for maintaining cellular structure and long-term health. Shorter transcripts, on the other hand, typically guide more immediate, short-term responses to cellular stress.

As cells age, they produce fewer long transcripts, a phenomenon known as "length-associated transcriptome imbalance." This effect is so pronounced that, in mouse models, nearly 80% of their tissues had an age-dependent decrease in long transcripts that was relatively consistent across different cell types. How come? Transcribing longer genes is a demanding task, making them more prone to degradation. RNA polymerase, the enzyme that reads DNA to create RNA, struggles more with longer genes as it contends with age-related DNA damage, chromatin compaction (a tighter packing of DNA), and declining cellular efficiency. These issues often result in incomplete or stalled transcripts.

By analyzing these age-related patterns in RNA expression, scientists have developed transcriptomic "clocks" to estimate biological age. While less mature than epigenetic clocks, transcriptomic clocks hold promise for capturing the dynamic nature of aging, offering a different lens to understand how our bodies adapt — or fail to adapt — over time.

Transcriptomics research is also opening new avenues for the study of cognitive decline, an unfortunate passenger of the aging process. Recent findings, for example, have uncovered a link between circulatory microRNAs (miRNAs) — tiny RNA molecules that regulate gene expression — and cognitive function, particularly in the context of dementia. By profiling over 500 well-expressed microRNAs in blood, scientists identified several strongly associated with cognitive health and dementia risk. Four of these emerged as potential biomarkers for both cognition and dementia.

While the exact role and mechanisms of these microRNAs are still unclear, we do have an inkling of what might be happening. For instance, they target genes expressed in critical brain regions like the hippocampus and cerebral cortex, areas integral to memory and cognitive processing. The microRNAs also appear to be involved in an important signaling pathway that helps neurons adjust their connections in response to new experiences — a process essential for learning and memory. This same pathway helps cells to send and receive chemical signals that coordinate their activities, ensuring the brain works as a cohesive unit. These processes are vital for maintaining cognitive health and adapting to changes in the environment. Subtle shifts in the activity of these microRNAs, then, can ripple across the brain's systems, potentially leading to cognitive decline.

What makes these findings so promising is the stability of microRNAs in bodily fluids, such as blood, making them excellent candidates for non-invasive biomarkers. By detecting and monitoring them, researchers could develop tools to identify individuals at risk of cognitive decline long before symptoms appear, opening the doors for early intervention.

Beyond tracking aging, transcriptomics as a whole represents a fertile field for the identification of new therapeutic targets. By pinpointing specific genes or pathways that change with age, researchers can design drugs or interventions to modulate these processes. For instance, if a certain RNA molecule becomes overactive in older cells, silencing that molecule might help restore balance and prevent disease. Similarly, understanding how age affects RNA's role in processes like protein synthesis or stress response can lead to innovations in treating age-related conditions.

## Challenges and Limitations

Despite its potential, transcriptomics is not without challenges. One significant limitation is the transient nature of RNA. Unlike DNA, which remains relatively stable, RNA molecules are short-lived and highly responsive to environmental and cellular conditions. This makes transcriptomic data inherently variable and context-dependent, complicating efforts to draw universal conclusions.

Another challenge lies in distinguishing cause from effect. Are the changes observed in RNA expression driving aging, or are they simply a consequence of it? For instance, the observed decline in long RNA transcripts with age could reflect an underlying issue like transcriptional stress or DNA damage, rather than being a primary driver of aging. This should be familiar to you from our discussion of epigenetic clocks, which share similar shortcomings.

Finally, transcriptomics faces technical hurdles. High-throughput RNA sequencing generates vast amounts of data, requiring sophisticated computational tools to analyze and interpret. Even with advanced algorithms, distinguishing meaningful patterns from noise can be daunting, particularly when studying such multi-faceted traits like aging.

## Proteomics: The Machinery of Life

Proteomics dives deeper into the functional machinery of cells by studying proteins — the molecules responsible for virtually all cellular activities. Unlike RNA, which serves as a set of instructions, proteins are the workers that build, repair, and regulate our bodies. As we age, our proteins tell a story. Their levels, interactions, and even their shapes change, reflecting how well—or poorly—our bodies are coping with time.

Plasma proteomics, which focuses on proteins in the blood, has identified specific molecules that act like signposts for aging. One standout is growth differentiation factor 15 (GDF15), often called the "aging protein." High levels of GDF15 have been linked to chronic diseases like heart failure and dementia. In fact, middle-aged adults with high levels of GDF15 tend to perform much more poorly on tests measuring focus, attention, and executive functioning.

Another brain-related protein, brevican (BCAN), has also been pinpointed as a signal for the onset of cognitive decline. Brevican is a key component of the brain's extracellular matrix (ECM), which plays a vital role in maintaining its structure. Although the nuances are still being uncovered, researchers suspect that fluctuations in brevican can disrupt the function of the extracellular matrix, potentially upsetting the balance between providing structural support and allowing for synaptic remodeling — an ongoing process where connections between neurons are strengthened, weakened, or reorganized. This remodeling is crucial for synaptic activity, the electrical and chemical communication between neurons that underpins learning, memory, and overall brain function. It goes without saying that disruption of these processes isn't the best thing for our brains.

Discoveries of this type could lead to earlier diagnoses of conditions like Alzheimer's and new therapies to slow their progression. When it comes to dementia, and most age-related diseases, early detection is critical to slowing its advance. And while we still lack clear treatments — let alone a cure — early intervention can help manage, and even reverse, symptoms.

What makes proteomics especially exciting is its ability to capture the here and now. Unlike your DNA, which stays the same throughout life, your proteins are constantly changing. They respond to what you eat, how you exercise, and even the stress you experience. This means proteomic markers can track the real-time effects of aging and, potentially, the impact of lifestyle changes or medical treatments.

But the sheer complexity of the proteome —the complete set of proteins in the body— is both its strength and its obstacle. Since proteins are constantly modified and influenced by their environment, they can be tricky to interpret. When we see changes in protein levels, are they a direct result of aging, or are they influenced by disease or other external factors? And while high-tech tools like mass spectrometry have revolutionized the field, they're still expensive and require expert handling, which can limit broader use.

Still, the potential is enormous. Down the road, a simple blood test could reveal everything from your biological age to the exact proteins contributing to any decline. Armed with this information, doctors could tailor treatments to your unique molecular profile.

∿ﾟ

## Multi-Omics: The Whole Symphony

While each omics field provides valuable insights, the real power lies in combining them. Multi-omics approaches integrate data from genomics, transcriptomics, and proteomics to paint a comprehensive picture of aging. This integration allows researchers to identify connections between molecular changes that would be invisible in isolated datasets.

For example, just recently scientists uncovered a striking insight into the nature of aging: it doesn't progress in a smooth, linear fashion. Instead, aging appears to occur in waves, with significant molecular and biological shifts peaking around two key ages: 40 and 60. These findings come from a comprehensive multi-omics study tracking over 100 participants across several years. By analyzing data from various molecular layers, the study identified distinct patterns of change tied to these age thresholds.

At the first peak, around 40, the focus is on metabolism. Changes in lipid and alcohol metabolism, as well as shifts in cardiovascular health markers, highlight the body's transition into midlife. By the second peak, at 60, immune system dysregulation takes center stage, alongside noticeable declines in kidney and muscle function. These crests signal critical moments when the risk of age-related diseases like cardiovascular conditions and neurodegeneration may accelerate.

~•

## Mapping the Future of Aging Research

Omics research is revolutionizing the study of aging by capturing the complexity of biological systems. Each field provides a unique lens for understanding the molecular shifts that drive aging and disease. And when combined, these fields offer an unprecedented opportunity to develop new biomarkers, interventions, and therapies. As technology advances, omics research may one day become part of routine healthcare, enabling clinicians to tailor treatments based on an individual's molecular profile.

~~

## Gait, Grip, and Balance: Physical Biomarkers of Aging

While the molecular world offers remarkable insights into the aging process, there's another important dimension: the physical signs of aging. Things like gait, grip strength, and balance, are more tangible and immediately observable than the biomarkers I previously discussed. After all, you can keep tabs on how your gait and how your balance are doing quite easily, but I'd be beyond impressed if you could gauge your body's complete proteome off the top of your head.

Despite being significantly less fine-grained, these bodily markers can still tell us a great deal about biological age — and this without access to a complex lab test. In a sense, it is precisely their weakness — lack of detail — that is also their strength, since it provides us with a way we can give ourselves a quick check up from the comforts of our homes.

## Gait Speed: The Rhythm of Aging

Walking may seem effortless, but it's a nuanced process requiring coordination between the brain, muscles, and joints. As we age, our way of walking, or gait, often slows — a change so consistent that researchers now view gait speed as one of the most reliable indicators of biological aging. Studies have shown that slower gait speed is linked to a higher risk of mortality, cardiovascular disease, and cognitive decline. In fact, for every quarter mile per hour (approximately) decrease in walking speed, there is an associated 21% increase in mortality risk. So, a drop in gait speed can sometimes predict health problems before they become clinically apparent.

The reasons behind this decline are multifaceted. Aging affects muscle strength, joint flexibility, and neural coordination — all critical components of walking. Additionally, diseases like arthritis or neuropathy can exacerbate these changes. But gait speed is more than just a marker of physical decline; it reflects overall vitality. For instance, someone with a quicker, more fluid gait is often better equipped to recover from illness or surgery than someone whose movements are slower and more hesitant.

Encouragingly, gait speed is not fixed. Exercise programs focused on strength, balance, and endurance can help improve our walking ability, even for the oldest among us. As is so often the case when it comes to aging, gait speed inhabits a two-faced role: one the one hand, it acts as a marker for the aging process, and on the other, it presents a potential site of intervention for reversing its effects.

## Grip Strength, More Than Just a Firm Handshake

If gait speed is a window into overall vitality, grip strength is a direct measure of physical power. Grip strength —simply how firmly someone can squeeze an object— has been widely studied as a marker of health and aging. Its significance might surprise you. Research has linked weaker grip strength with higher mortality risk, increased likelihood of developing chronic diseases, and even cognitive decline.

Why does grip strength matter so much? The answer lies in what it represents. A strong grip reflects robust muscle mass and function, which in turn signals overall physical resilience. Since muscle mass naturally declines with age, tracking grip strength offers a simple yet effective way to monitor this change. Moreover, weaker grip strength can indicate frailty, a condition characterized by reduced strength, endurance, and physiological function.

What's more, grip strength is easy to measure. A simple hand dynamometer can provide a quick assessment, making it a practical tool for researchers, healthcare providers, and you. Like gait speed, grip strength can be improved through targeted interventions, including resistance training and adequate protein intake.

## Watch Your Step! Balance and Stability

Balance is one of those abilities we often take for granted until it begins to fail. Poor balance increases the risk of falls, which are among the leading causes of injury and mortality in older adults. The ability to maintain balance depends on a complex interplay between sensory systems (vision, inner ear, proprioception), muscles, and the brain. Aging disrupts these systems, leading to slower reflexes, weaker muscles, and a diminished ability to sense the body's position in space.

Tests like standing on one leg or walking heel-to-toe are simple ways to assess balance, and they often reveal more than just physical limitations. For example, difficulty balancing may signal underlying neurological or cardiovascular issues. Interestingly, some studies have suggested that balance tests can even predict longevity. People who perform poorly on balance assessments are often at higher risk of mortality compared to their more stable peers.

But again, balance is an area where improvements are possible. Exercises like tai chi, yoga, and targeted balance training can strengthen the muscles and reflexes involved, reducing fall risk and improving overall stability.

## Everything Has Limitations

Despite their utility, physical markers have their limitations. For one, they can be influenced by factors unrelated to aging, such as injury, chronic illness, or even short-term fatigue. This makes it crucial to interpret these markers in context. On top of this, while physical tests are practical and low-cost, they don't provide the detailed molecular insights that omics research offers. Bridging this gap will require integrating physical markers with molecular data, creating a more holistic understanding of aging.

# CHAPTER 24

# Mending a Broken Heart: Medicine and Cardiovascular Health

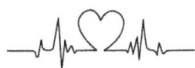

Heart disease continues to be the most common cause of illness and death in developed countries. As with many other conditions, it becomes increasingly prevalent the older we grow, making aging itself one of the strongest predictors of heart health. The statistics speak for themselves: nearly 40% of people between the ages of 40 and 59 have some form of heart disease, and this jumps to 75% in those aged 60-79. Meanwhile, in those aged 80 and older, a staggering 86% suffer from heart issues. Alongside this, hypertension — what most people call high blood pressure — is almost ubiquitous among older adults, affecting over 70% of men and nearly 78% of women aged 65-74.

How come there's such a sharp uptick in cardiovascular disease with age? Well, arteries lose their elasticity, stiffening like old rubber bands. This increases blood pressure and forces the heart to work harder. Meanwhile, the heart muscle itself becomes less efficient, pumping blood with a little less vigor. These changes are often subtle in the early stages, but over time, they can snowball into serious complications. So, the question isn't just how we slow this decline but how we reverse it — and yes, emerging research suggests we might be on the cusp of groundbreaking solutions.

## Established Therapies: A Pillar of Cardiovascular Care

Modern medicine's ability to treat cardiovascular disease is one of its most remarkable achievements. Decades of research, innovation, and clinical application have led to therapies that not only extend life but also dramatically improve its quality. From medications to surgical interventions, these treatments form the backbone of our fight against heart disease.

## The Evolution of Cardiovascular Medications

The development of cardiovascular drugs began with a deeper understanding of the mechanisms behind heart disease. In the 20th century, researchers identified high blood pressure and cholesterol as major contributors to heart attacks and strokes. This insight led to the development of two game-changing classes of drugs: antihypertensives and statins.

Antihypertensives, like ACE inhibitors and beta-blockers, revolutionized the treatment of high blood pressure. By relaxing blood vessels or slowing the heart rate, these medications reduce the strain on the cardiovascular system, significantly lowering the risk of heart attacks and strokes. Their widespread adoption has made conditions like hypertension — once a leading cause of premature death — manageable for millions worldwide.

Statins, introduced in the late 1980s, were another transformative advance. These drugs target cholesterol by blocking an enzyme involved in its production, leading to lower low-density lipoprotein (LDL) levels in the bloodstream. Statins not only prevent heart disease in at-risk individuals but also reduce the recurrence of heart attacks in those with existing conditions. Their impact is so profound that statins are now considered a cornerstone of preventive cardiology.

## Surgical Interventions

For those whose conditions are too advanced for medication alone, surgical interventions have offered lifesaving options. Coronary artery bypass grafting, developed in the 1960s, was one of the first procedures to restore blood flow to the heart by rerouting blocked arteries. Over time, advances in technology and surgical techniques have made the procedure safer and more effective.

Then, towards the latter half of the 1970s, angioplasty was introduced, offering a less invasive alternative. Using a small balloon to open clogged arteries, followed by the placement of a stent to keep them open, angioplasty quickly became a standard treatment for acute heart attacks. These procedures have dramatically improved survival rates, turning what were once fatal events into manageable medical crises.

## Devices

Implantable devices have also played a critical role in managing cardiovascular disease. Pacemakers, which regulate abnormal heart rhythms, and implantable cardioverter defibrillators (ICDs), which prevent sudden cardiac death, have saved countless lives. More recently, advancements like left ventricular assist devices (LVADs) have provided hope for patients with end-stage heart failure, serving as a bridge to heart transplants or as long-term therapy.

~

## Experimental Therapies: Pushing the Boundaries of Cardiovascular Medicine

While established treatments have transformed care, the really exciting stuff lies ahead of us; researchers continue to push the boundaries of what's possible. Emerging therapies aim not just to manage symptoms but to address the root causes of cardiovascular aging.

~~◦

## Targeting Cellular Senescence

Remember those senescent cells I talked about in earlier chapters, the ones that are often described as the "zombies" of the cellular world? As a refresher, these are cells that stop dividing but refuse to die, lingering in tissues where they release a mix of inflammatory molecules and enzymes. But they aren't all bad: in small amounts, this process serves a protective role by assisting in wound repair and by preventing damaged cells from turning cancerous. However, when senescent cells accumulate, as they often do with age, their presence becomes toxic, driving inflammation and tissue dysfunction.

### The Burden of Senescence in Cardiovascular Health

Senescence is implicated in almost every aspect of cardiovascular aging, from the stiffening of arteries to the progression of heart failure. Endothelial cells, which line the inner walls of blood vessels, are especially vulnerable. When they become senescent, they lose their ability to regulate blood flow, allowing plaques to form along the vessel walls and increasing the risk of atherosclerosis.

Similarly, senescent vascular smooth muscle cells destabilize these plaques, raising the likelihood of heart attack or stroke. Even cardiac fibroblasts, which maintain the structural integrity of the heart, can turn senescent, contributing to myocardial fibrosis — a condition that stiffens the heart and impairs its ability to pump blood effectively.

Recent studies also point to senescence as a key player in microvascular dysfunction, which affects the tiny blood vessels that nourish the heart and other tissues. This dysfunction can lead to chronic ischemia, a condition where tissues don't receive enough oxygen, further exacerbating cardiovascular decline.

## Senolytics: Eliminating Senescence

The discovery of senolytics — compounds that selectively eliminate senescent cells — has brought new hope to the field of geroscience. Drugs like dasatinib and quercetin have shown remarkable results in preclinical models, effectively reducing senescent cell burden and reversing some signs of cardiovascular aging. For example, animal studies have demonstrated that senolytics can restore vascular elasticity, reduce inflammation, and even improve heart function. These functional improvements extended to the animals' ability to withstand cardiovascular stress, suggesting that senolytics could play a preventative role as well as a therapeutic one.

Beyond the heart, senolytics have shown promise in addressing systemic inflammation, which is a serious contributor to cardiovascular decline. By reducing inflammatory signals, these compounds might be able to help us break the vicious cycle of chronic inflammation and tissue damage.

## Challenges, Precision, and Personalization

The current generation of senolytics is only the beginning. Future therapies will refine the approach, targeting specific types of senescent cells while sparing others. This precision is crucial, as not all senescent cells are harmful. For example, senescent cells in certain contexts help resolve fibrosis and support tissue regeneration. Eliminating these cells indiscriminately could have unintended consequences, including delayed recovery from injuries or weakened defenses against cancer.

This concern is even more pronounced when it comes to cells that naturally do not divide. Neurons, for instance, don't divide like other cells, yet they still rely on pathways that help them survive stress and damage. These "pro-survival pathways" act like life-support systems, keeping neurons functional even under tough conditions. Unfortunately, senolytics are built to target those same pathways because senescent cells often use them as a crutch to evade natural cell death. The result? Senolytics can't always tell the difference between a damaged, senescent cell and a perfectly healthy, non-dividing neuron — they see the same survival signals and may mistakenly attack. Part of the issue is that we do not yet have a universal "fingerprint" to identify senescent cells, increasing the risk of friendly fire.

Some emerging strategies, like "senomorphics," aim to bypass these worries. Senomorphics are compounds that don't kill senescent cells but instead suppress their harmful activity. By modulating rather than eradicating these cells, they could provide a safer alternative, minimizing risks while retaining the protective roles of senescence where they are needed.

Despite the excitement, translating senolytics into clinical practice remains a daunting task. Human aging is vastly more complex than animal models, and senolytics that work in mice may not have the same efficacy or safety profile in humans. Some early trials have raised concerns about potential side effects, such as off-target toxicity and impacts on platelet function. Platelets are the tiny cell fragments in your blood responsible for clotting and preventing excessive bleeding. By disrupting platelet function, some senolytics increase the risk of uncontrolled bleeding or bruising. This makes them a double-edged sword: while effective at clearing senescent cells, their impact on essential blood components means we need to move with caution.

What's more, questions remain about how to best deliver these therapies. Senolytics often require careful dosing schedules to avoid unintended harm, and the development of biomarkers to identify which patients would benefit most is still in progress. Advances in drug delivery systems — such as nanoparticles that target senescent cells more precisely — could help overcome such challenges, but for now these, too, are still largely experimental.

~⁃

## Gene Therapy and CRISPR: The Future of Cardiovascular Medicine?

The advent of gene therapy and CRISPR-based technologies marks a transformative era in cardiovascular medicine. At its core, gene therapy aims to correct or change genetic elements to treat or prevent disease, offering hope for conditions previously deemed incurable. Meanwhile, CRISPR (Clustered Regularly Interspaced

Short Palindromic Repeats) represents a powerful tool for precisely editing the genome, allowing for unprecedented interventions in both inherited and acquired heart disorders.

## Gene Therapy: Improving Genetic Instructions

Gene therapy works by delivering new or modified genes into a patient's cells to correct genetic errors or bolster cellular function. Think of it as editing a faulty instruction manual: if a key page is missing or has a mistake, gene therapy fills in the gaps with the correct information.

One of the earliest cardiovascular applications involved the *SERCA2a* gene, which regulates calcium in heart muscle cells. In heart failure, this mechanism often breaks down, leading to impaired pumping ability. To tackle the problem, researchers delivered a working copy of the *SERCA2a* gene directly into heart cells, using a harmless virus, called a viral vector, as a delivery vehicle. This works like a tiny courier service: the virus is engineered to carry the healthy gene into the cells without causing harm. Once inside, the gene instructs the cells to produce the proteins needed to restore normal calcium regulation. Although the trial yielded mixed results, it paved the way for more refined approaches.

Amongst these newer approaches is "therapeutic angiogenesis," which is a complicated term for a pretty simple idea: artificially kickstarting the growth of new blood vessels. As the population ages and survival rates improve for patients with coronary artery disease, a growing number of individuals find themselves grappling with refractory angina — persistent chest pain caused by blocked arteries that doesn't respond to standard medical treatments. These unlucky patients, often referred to as having "no-option" angina, have exhausted conventional interventions like bypass surgery or stent placement, leaving them with few, if any, therapeutic avenues. Enter therapeutic angiogenesis. By introducing genes that are intimately linked to blood-vessel growth — like *VEGF* (vascular endothelial growth factor) — this therapy effectively creates new, alternative pathways for blood flow. It's a nifty workaround to a blockade: if you can't go through, just go around. And indeed, it's been helping many of these patients find much-needed relief.

Another new gene therapy for cardiovascular health focuses on pericytes, which are specialized cells that maintain blood vessel structure and function. As we age, pericytes lose their effectiveness, leading to weaker blood vessels and poorer heart performance. But there's a lucky set of people who carry a particular gene variant — *LAV-BPIFB4*— that protects heart health by more effectively supporting pericytes in their duties. Indeed, this gene variant is common amongst the superheroes of aging, centenarians. And in general, individuals carrying this variant exhibit fewer cardiovascular complications and better heart health even into old age.

Scientists have started to take note, exploring whether this gene could be leveraged for a longevity boost in those of us who did not win the lottery. In a recent study, for instance, researchers introduced the *LAV-BPIFB4* gene into the hearts of elderly mice. The result? The gene variant rewound markers of biological heart aging by the equivalent of more than 10 human years. And the effects weren't restricted to elderly mice: introducing the gene in middle age helped stop the decline of heart function, effectively nipping it in the bud.

While these initial trials used mouse models, there's reason to believe the benefits may carry over to us. The same researchers exposed human heart cells from patients with severe heart failure to the longevity gene. Impressively, these cells, which typically show signs of aging and reduced functionality, regained their ability to support vascular networks after exposure to *LAV-BPIFB4*. In fact, there were even hints of the same kind of "reverse aging" that they had seen in the mouse models, with the cells beginning to resemble those from healthier, younger hearts.

## CRISPR: Molecular Scissors

While gene therapy introduces new instructions, CRISPR takes it a step further: it allows scientists to directly edit the DNA itself. This revolutionary gene-editing tool acts like a pair of "molecular scissors," capable of cutting DNA at precise locations. The CRISPR system includes two main components: the Cas9 protein, which makes the cut, and a guide RNA, which directs Cas9 to the specific DNA sequence to be edited. Think of it as a search-and-replace function for the genome, where scientists can find problematic genes and fix them.

### Headway in the Fight Against Cholesterol

Advances in CRISPR technology have led to even more refined techniques, such as single-letter base editing. Traditional CRISPR cuts the DNA, which triggers the cell's repair mechanisms to replace or fix the damaged segment. However, base editing skips the cutting step altogether. Instead, it chemically modifies a single DNA letter (a base) to correct a mutation — like replacing a typo in a long text without disrupting the surrounding words. This approach is gentler and reduces the risk of unintended changes, known as off-target effects, and has opened up exciting possibilities for treating inherited cardiovascular diseases.

In fact, this technique was just recently used to successfully cure familial hypercholesterolemia, a condition where dangerously high cholesterol levels are passed down through families due to inherited genetic mutations. This occurs because certain variants of the *PCSK9* gene fail to regulate cholesterol properly, leading to a buildup of LDL, or "bad cholesterol," in the bloodstream.

For individuals with the more common heterozygous form of the condition, where one faulty gene is inherited, life expectancy can be shortened by 20 to 30 years compared to the general population. In fact, without treatment, only about one in five men with familial hypercholesterolemia reach the age of 70. The rarer and more severe homozygous form is even more devastating. In this case, people inherit harmful variants from both parents, and without intervention, life expectancy averages just 30 years, with many dying before the age of 20.

In early human trials, a team of researchers used CRISPR base editing to modify the *PCSK9* genes in individuals with the heritable condition. The results were truly remarkable. By altering a single DNA letter, they were able to permanently reduce LDL cholesterol levels by up to 55%.

But here's the exciting part: this treatment isn't limited to people with familial hypercholesterolemia. The mechanism by which *PCSK9* regulates cholesterol applies universally, meaning the same approach could benefit anyone struggling with high LDL cholesterol, even if they don't have the condition. Studies in mice with normal genetics have already shown that editing PCSK9 reduces both plasma PCSK9 levels and cholesterol, pointing to a broad application for this therapy. Similarly, humans with natural loss-of-function mutations in *PCSK9* enjoy significantly lower LDL cholesterol levels and reduced cardiovascular risk, acting as a "proof of principle" for the potential benefits of this pathway.

By permanently switching off *PCSK9* in the liver, base editing offers a one-and-done solution to lower cholesterol and reduce the risk of heart attacks and strokes. For millions of people currently relying on daily medications like statins, this breakthrough could represent a revolutionary shift in how we manage cardiovascular health, replacing lifelong drug regimens with a single treatment designed to protect the heart for decades.

## Challenges and Ethical Considerations

Despite representing huge advances in medicine, CRISPR and gene therapy do come with their share of hurdles. Effective delivery of these technologies remains a central challenge. For treatments to work, the genetic editing tools — whether they're CRISPR molecules or therapeutic genes — must reach the right cells in the right tissues without causing unintended effects elsewhere in the body. To achieve this, researchers often use viral vectors, such as adeno-associated viruses (AAVs). As previously mentioned, these viruses act as delivery vehicles, engineered to carry therapeutic material into the targeted cells.

But the use of viral vectors is not entirely without risks. Some patients may experience immune responses, where the body's defense system attacks the viral delivery mechanism, reducing the treatment's effectiveness and potentially causing harmful inflammation. Adding to this, there's the issue of off-target effects —

when the editing tools mistakenly alter DNA sequences outside the intended target. These unintended edits could disrupt critical genes, leading to unforeseen complications, including cancer. To mitigate these risks, scientists are exploring alternative delivery systems, such as lipid nanoparticles, which may offer greater precision and lower the likelihood of immune reactions. If that name rings a bell, that's because the mRNA vaccines against COVID-19 made use of the same nanoparticle approach.

Beyond technical challenges, there are also serious ethical implications of CRISPR-based treatments that demand careful consideration. One of the most contentious issues is the prospect of germline editing. This involves making genetic changes to eggs, sperm, or embryos, which are then passed down to future generations. While germline editing could, in theory, eliminate inherited diseases, it should give us pause. What happens if unintended mutations are passed on? Could this technology lead to a future of "designer babies," where genetic traits are selected for non-medical reasons, further deepening societal inequalities?

Unfortunately, cost is another critical factor. Gene therapies and CRISPR-based treatments are among the most expensive medical interventions ever developed. This "paywall" forces us to consider the implications on healthcare disparities; might the treatments exacerbate existing gaps in access, limiting their availability to only the wealthiest patients or countries? If these technologies are to fulfill their promise of revolutionizing medicine, we need to develop strategies to make them affordable and accessible to all, not just a privileged few.

Despite these challenges, the field continues to advance, with researchers and policymakers working to address the various concerns. For one, regulatory frameworks are being refined to ensure that safety and ethical standards keep pace with advances. Meanwhile, ongoing research into alternative delivery systems and cost-effective production methods holds promise for overcoming many of the financial obstacles. As with any transformative technology, the path forward requires balancing innovation with responsibility.

~

## Stem Cells and Tissue Engineering: Regenerating Tired Hearts

The heart is an extraordinary organ, stubbornly pumping blood through our bodies, day and night, from birth to death. Yet, for all its strength, the adult human heart has a critical weakness: it struggles to repair itself after injury. Unlike the skin, which regenerates new cells to heal a wound, or the liver, which can regrow even after substantial damage, the heart has almost no capacity for regeneration. Why?

The answer lies in the heart's cellular makeup. Most of the heart's muscle cells, called cardiomyocytes, are formed before birth and during early development. By adulthood, these cells stop dividing and enter a state of stasis. This means that, after an injury like a heart attack, where millions of cardiomyocytes die due to lack of oxygen, the heart can't replace them. Instead, scar tissue forms — a patchwork repair that compromises the heart's ability to pump blood efficiently.

A key factor in our hearts' inability to repair itself is the role of the extracellular matrix, a structural network surrounding heart cells that becomes increasingly rigid with age. This stiffness inhibits the ability of remaining cardiomyocytes to divide and replace damaged tissue.

To top things off, as our heart cells grow older they experience a significant drop in the number of nuclear pores — structures that act as communication highways between the information center of the cell and the rest of the cell. By reducing crosstalk between heart cells and their surroundings, the heart shields itself from harmful stress signals, such as those caused by high blood pressure. But, this protective strategy comes with a trade-off: it also blocks the regenerative signals that could help repair damaged heart tissue.

Much to our misfortune, these regenerative shortfalls become increasingly problematic as we age. Much to our fortune, we're finding strategies to fight back. While gene therapy and CRISPR take action at the genetic level, there are other, more "fleshy" approaches to healing aging and damaged cardiovascular systems.

## Stem Cells: A Blank Slate

Pluripotent stem cells are a marvel of biology, serving as the foundation from which all the diverse cells in the human body arise. The discovery of their existence transformed our understanding of development and regeneration, opening doors to revolutionary medical possibilities.

The journey began with studies of embryonic development, where researchers observed that cells in the early embryo could give rise to every tissue type in the body — skin, muscle, nerves, and more. These cells, termed pluripotent, are like a blank slate, equipped with the potential to become any specialized cell depending on the signals they receive. In a sense, they act as the architects of our development, orchestrating the formation of our organs and systems.

Then, back in 2006, the field enjoyed a massive breakthrough: a Japanese scientist called Dr. Shinya Yamanaka discovered that it was possible to turn back the clock on adult cells. By introducing specific genetic factors, he and his team were able to reprogram ordinary somatic cells — like skin or blood cells — into induced pluripotent stem cells (iPSCs). These induced stem cells regain the same versatility as embryonic stem cells, capable of transforming into any cell type. This discovery not only circumvented the ethical concerns surrounding embryonic stem cell use but also created new possibilities for regenerative medicine, allowing scientists to generate patient-specific stem cells for research and therapy.

It didn't take long for the medical community to start thinking of ways to co-opt the new technology towards practical purposes. Now, a little less than twenty years later, we are starting to feel the benefits of their hard work.

In preclinical studies, mesenchymal stem cells derived from bone marrow or adipose tissue have demonstrated significant therapeutic benefits. When injected directly into damaged heart tissue, these cells cut down inflammation, boost the formation of new blood vessels, and promote the repair of cardiac muscles. In patients with ischemic heart failure — a condition where the heart struggles to pump blood efficiently due to damage caused by reduced blood flow or oxygen supply — stem cells have revamped the heart's pumping ability and reduced biomarkers of heart stress.

Stem-cell therapy has also proven itself useful in improving quality of life for patients with advanced heart failure. In one of the largest clinical trials of its kind, researchers at the Mayo Clinic found that patients receiving stem cells fine-tuned for heart repair experienced reduced daily burdens compared to those relying solely on standard treatments; breathing became easier, they were less fatigued than usual, their legs less swollen, and they were even able to incorporate more exercise back into their life. The therapy also lowered rates of death and hospitalization, suggesting it could offer both physical and emotional benefits for individuals living with heart failure.

As people live longer, they often face chronic conditions that significantly impact their quality of life, turning years of extended life expectancy into years marked by fatigue, physical limitation, and emotional strain. In this context, stem-cell-based therapy emerges as a beacon of hope. Dr. Andre Terzic, a leading cardiovascular researcher, emphasizes the promise of regenerative medicine in transforming how we approach heart failure. Stem-cell therapies, he notes, provide sustained benefits, helping patients regain not just the ability to perform daily activities but also a renewed sense of vitality.

## Tissue Engineering: Organic Scaffolding

Tissue engineering stands out as a cutting-edge area of regenerative medicine, aiming to rebuild or replace damaged tissues by combining living cells with advanced materials and engineering techniques. While stem-cell therapies typically involve injecting individual cells into the body to promote healing, tissue engineering takes a more structured approach. It focuses on creating three-dimensional (3D) constructs designed to replicate the form and function of the original tissue. These constructs often include biomaterial scaffolds, which act like a framework, providing support for cells as they grow, mature, and integrate seamlessly with the body's existing tissues.

## Regenerating the Heart After Damage

Heart attacks leave portions of the heart scarred and unable to contract effectively. Advances in tissue engineering are allowing us to address this; researchers have developed engineered cardiac tissues composed of the various cells that make up our heart. These cells, which are often derived from human pluripotent stem cells, are carefully organized into three-dimensional constructs that mimic the structure of native heart tissue. Once transplanted, the engineered tissues can integrate with the heart of their new host, improving its ability to pump blood while reducing the scarring that stiffens and weakens the heart.

## Understanding Disease Through Engineered Models

Tissue engineering is also revolutionizing our understanding of the heart by creating "organs on a chip" that we can study in real-time. Picture this: a small blood sample from a patient with a heart condition is reprogrammed into pluripotent stem cells. These cells are then coaxed, with the help of biomaterial scaffolds, to become heart cells that mimic the patient's unique biology. The result is a living, beating heart model in a lab — a tool that allows scientists to study the disease's behavior, explore its mechanisms, and test potential treatments. This deeply personalized approach not only enhances our ability to predict how a patient might respond to therapies but also provides an ethical alternative to animal testing. By bridging the gap between laboratory discovery and real-world application, tissue engineering is ushering in a paradigm shift in organ research.

## The Holy Grail: Growing Replacement Organs

The discussion of stem cells and of tissue engineering leads us to the "holy grail" of regenerative medicine: lab-grown organs. While fixing something is a good first step, sometimes you reach a point where the only remaining option is to replace it entirely. The same holds true of organic tissue and organs — when worse comes to worst, there's nothing left for us but to attempt an organ transplant. But, despite all of our advances, this remains a fraught affair. You see, our immune system is quite picky; it doesn't like anything that isn't clearly its own. This includes foreign organs (even if these organs are being introduced with the intent of helping to replace an unsalvageable organ). Our body doesn't care about intent, foreign is foreign. And so, it begins rejecting the new organs. This leads to all kinds of complications and auto-immune concerns.

So, how do we circumvent these issues? Well, what could be better than replacing one of your organs with another one of *your* organs. Except, you know, one grown in a lab using your stem cells. Voila, no more rejection issues. A vision of on-demand organ replacement that could one day eradicate waiting lists for transplants and eliminate the risk of rejection.

Or so the idea goes. Unfortunately, we're still a ways off from making it reality — but there are grounds for excitement.

### *A Brief History of Lab-Grown Organs*

The journey began with relatively simple structures. In the 1990s, researchers achieved early success with tissues like skin and cartilage, which are less complex and more forgiving in their structural requirements. The real game-changer came in the mid-2000s with the discovery of induced pluripotent stem cells, which provided a versatile and ethical source of stem cells capable of differentiating into any cell type. Combined with advancements in 3D cell culture techniques and biomaterials, scientists began to tackle more complex tissue constructs.

By the early 2010s, the focus shifted toward creating organoids — miniature versions of organs grown from stem cells. These organoids, while small and incomplete, replicate many of the key features of organs like the brain, intestine, lung, and liver. They have proven invaluable for modeling diseases, testing drugs, and deepening our understanding of organ development.

Meanwhile, breakthroughs in bioprinting, which involves 3D printing living cells into tissue-like structures, has brought new hope for growing larger, functional organs. The printing process begins with a detailed blueprint, often derived from imaging technologies like MRI or CT scans, which maps out the organ or tissue's design. Using bioinks — a mixture of cells and supportive materials like hydrogels — the printer deposits these components layer by layer. The bioink not only positions the cells but also provides a supportive environment, promoting cell survival and growth. Recent advances have accelerated the printing process and improved resolution, bringing researchers closer to producing full-sized organs.

Decellularized scaffolds take a different yet complementary approach by using the extracellular matrix (ECM) of donor organs that are no longer viable for transplantation. These organs are stripped of their original cells, leaving behind a scaffold of proteins and fibers that retain the organ's shape and vascular pathways. This template is then repopulated with patient-specific cells, offering a framework for building new tissue.

## *Where We Are Today*

Despite remarkable progress, the creation of full-sized, fully functional organs remains elusive. Scientists can now bioprint simple structures like blood vessels and muscle tissue, and organoids are being used widely in research. However, the leap from small-scale models to transplant-ready organs faces daunting challenges.

One of the most significant hurdles is "vascularization" — creating the infinitely complex blood vessel networks required to sustain large tissues. Without a robust vascular system, lab-grown organs cannot survive or function when transplanted into a living body. Similarly, replicating the complexity of organs like the heart or liver, with their specialized cells and intricate architecture, remains a monumental task. Scalability is another challenge; while organoids are impressive, scaling them into functional, full-sized organs is a logistical and biological puzzle.

An additional factor that requires addressing is ensuring that lab-grown organs can perform all the necessary functions of their natural counterparts — such as filtering toxins in a liver or pumping blood in a heart.

### *What Lies Ahead?*

The future of lab-grown organs lies in integrating multiple approaches and technologies. Continued innovation in bioprinting promises to improve the structural and functional fidelity of engineered organs. Similarly, combining organoid technology with bioprinting and scaffold-based methods could pave the way for more complex structures.

Another possible direction involves interspecies chimeras. That is, growing human organs inside animal hosts, such as pigs. While this approach could overcome some challenges, it raises significant ethical concerns about the extent of human-animal integration and the moral implications of creating chimeric beings.

Although fully functional lab-grown organs are still on the horizon, the progress made so far is already transforming medicine. I speculate that, in a few more decades, patients may no longer face the agonizing uncertainty of waiting for a donor organ, as regenerative medicine will begin to fulfill its promise to heal and restore at an unprecedented scale.

# CHAPTER 25

# Strong Muscles, Solid Bones: Medicine and Musculoskeletal Health

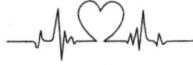

W hen we think about the hazards of aging, heart disease or cancer probably come to mind first. But there's another, quieter threat that impacts just as many lives — fractures caused by weakened bones and muscles. A hip fracture in an elderly adult, for example, can be more fatal than many types of cancer, with survival rates dropping below 50% in the first five years post-fracture. The first month after such an injury is especially critical, with complications from immobility and underlying frailty driving the sharpest decline in survival.

The takeaway is crystal clear: the integrity of our musculoskeletal system is central to aging well. Our bones and muscles form the scaffolding of our bodies, allowing us to move, balance, and maintain independence. Yet, as we age, this system undergoes dramatic changes. Bones lose density, muscles weaken, and injuries that might have been minor in youth become devastating in older age.

Physical activity aside — which continues to be the best way of keeping muscles strong and bones dense — cutting-edge science is also playing its part in challenging the inevitability of musculoskeletal decline. From therapies aimed at reversing muscle loss to advances in bone regeneration, researchers are helping us reimagine what it means to grow older. Here, we take a look at some

195

of these breakthroughs, starting with sarcopenia — our fight against muscle loss — and moving to osteoporosis, where we delve into the frontier of bone health innovations.

~♪

## Sarcopenia: Age-Related Muscle Loss

As we age, muscles that once powered us through hikes, dances, and daily routines begin to shrink and lose their strength; after our 30th birthday, we lose 3% to 5% of our muscle mass every decade. With time, this risks making even the simplest tasks feel daunting. This age-related loss of muscle is known as sarcopenia, and it affects millions of older adults worldwide. profoundly impacts their independence and their quality of life. It's more than just a nuisance; sarcopenia increases the risk of falls, fractures, and hospitalizations, casting a shadow over what should be vibrant later years.

But science is fighting back. The quest to combat sarcopenia has become a cornerstone of geroscience, with researchers exploring two complementary approaches. The first seeks to mimic the benefits of exercise — essentially bottling the molecular magic of movement for those unable to engage in regular physical activity. The second aims to directly rejuvenate and regenerate muscle tissue, restoring strength from within.

## Exercise in a Pill?

Regular exercise remains the ultimate prescription for keeping your muscles strong, and your body healthy. But what about those who can't engage in physical activity due to their age, chronic illness, or disability? For this population, science has been exploring a tantalizing alternative: so-called "exercise mimetics," compounds that aim to replicate the molecular effects of exercise without requiring a single step on the treadmill. These compounds tap into the same pathways activated during physical activity, offering hope to those of us for whom exercise is not an option.

A key breakthrough in this approach involves exerkines, a class of signaling molecules released by muscles during exercise. These proteins act as messengers, triggering systemic changes that benefit everything from glucose metabolism to heart health. By mimicking the action of exerkines, researchers have identified compounds that could simulate the effects of a workout at the cellular level.

Take AICAR, for instance. This compound works by activating an enzyme known as AMP-activated protein kinase (AMPK), often described as the body's energy sensor. When energy levels drop — such as during exercise — AMPK is triggered, prompting cells to burn stored fat and improve glucose uptake. AICAR essentially flips this same metabolic switch, boosting both the number and activity of our mitochondria. This uptick in mitochondria has been associated with improved endurance in preclinical studies. For individuals unable to engage in exercise, such a compound could offer a pathway to some of the same health benefits.

It is worth noting, however, that these findings remain in their preliminary stages, and not all research agrees on its benefits. Some studies suggest that AICAR's effects on mitochondria may be less pronounced than hoped, while others raise concerns about possible side effects. Overactivating AMPK or triggering it in the wrong tissue, for instance, might unintentionally interfere with the cell division process, which is critical for staying healthy (and just alive, for that matter). What's more, the natural buildup of AICAR has been linked to certain metabolic disorders in humans, highlighting the caution needed when targeting these pathways for therapeutic purposes. So, while promising, AICAR represents an as-yet uncertain avenue.

Luckily, we have other contenders. Sirtuins are a family of proteins that have a better safety profile and are still just as promising when it comes to improving mitochondrial health. Think of them as molecular efficiency experts, ensuring mitochondria function smoothly even under the pressures of aging. By activating specific enzymes, they help cells fend off damage and optimize energy use. Early research suggests that boosting sirtuin activity could help counteract the mitochondrial decline linked to sarcopenia, possibly reversing some of its damaging effects.

Another approach involves PPARδ activators — I know the name, with all its letters and symbols, is uninviting, but bear with me. PPARδ is a protein that regulates the expression of genes involved in fat metabolism. It plays a crucial role in determining muscle fiber type. Activating the protein encourages the development of slow-twitch muscle fibers, which are more efficient at using oxygen and are associated with improved endurance. By promoting this shift, PPARδ activators could enhance muscle composition and improve metabolic health in individuals struggling with muscle decline due to aging or disease.

The science behind exercise mimetics also underscores a broader principle: the body's response to movement is not an all-or-nothing process. By targeting specific pathways, researchers can isolate and replicate individual benefits of exercise, such as improved insulin sensitivity or enhanced mitochondrial function.

Where does all of this leave us? Instead of viewing physical activity as the sole means of improving muscle health, exercise mimetics open the door to drugs that replicate these effects. While for now I don't think these treatments can replace the holistic benefits of actual movement — including mental health and improved balance — they offer an invaluable option for those who face significant barriers to traditional exercise. With a little more research, these compounds could bridge the gap between possibility and limitation.

## (Re)Generating Muscle: The Stem-Cell Approach

For the most part, muscle tissue is exceptionally capable of repairing itself. Think of the last time you exercised. You were probably sore for a day or two afterward, but this soon went away. That's evidence of muscle repairing itself in real time. Similarly, most muscular injuries require little to no medical intervention — given rest and time, they heal by themselves.

But in rare cases, including severe muscle injuries, certain genetic diseases, and especially age-related muscle loss, the usual regenerative magic fails. Here, we need a therapeutic approach to fall back on, one that can pick up the slack when our muscles no longer can.

Enter stem-cell therapies. These aim to harness stem cells to restore what aging has taken away, offering a lifeline to muscles struggling to regenerate. At the forefront of this effort are two distinct approaches: 1) rejuvenating the muscle-specific stem cells that are already present in our bodies, and 2) introducing new stem cells derived from advanced technologies like human-induced pluripotent stem cells. Both strategies hold tremendous promise, but they also face significant hurdles that researchers are racing to overcome.

## Rejuvenation

At the heart of the muscle-regeneration approach are satellite cells, specialized muscle stem cells that remain dormant until injury activates them. These cells are vital for repairing damaged muscle and replenishing its structure. However, over a lifetime, satellite cells lose their vigor. They decline in both number and function, accumulating intrinsic defects that impair their ability to self-renew or respond to repair signals. This breakdown in function underpins sarcopenia, leaving aging muscles more prone to weakness and wasting.

Advances in laboratory techniques have provided a glimpse of what's possible. Researchers have shown that manipulating specific "signaling channels" in aged satellite cells can restore their regenerative potential. For instance, there's a channel that becomes hyperactive in aging cells. Targeting this channel can reawaken dormant regenerative abilities — a little like a loud alarm clock that gets you up and moving first thing in the morning. Coupled with biomaterials like hydrogels, which mimic the elasticity of young muscle tissue, these rejuvenated cells have been able to restore muscle strength in experimental models. Although these are only baby steps for now, they are testament that the approach, at least in theory, works.

Another intriguing area of research looks at how factors in the bloodstream affect muscle stem cells. Experiments in animals have shown that connecting the blood circulation of a younger and an older animal can refresh aging cells. This discovery has sparked interest in identifying specific "youth factors" in young blood, such as a protein called GDF11, which may hold the key to reactivating muscle stem cells and boosting regeneration. Of course, this comes with a host of ethical considerations — I'll leave you to come up with the relevant dystopian scenarios that a lack of oversight and regulation could lead to.

## Replacement

When rejuvenation fails, we have to look toward replacement. Stem cell therapy may seem like an obvious option for dealing with muscle loss: just replace old muscle stem cells struggling to perform their job with new ones. While this sounds great in theory, it has proven quite difficult in practice. The main issue is that the transplanted muscle stem cells fail to integrate into the muscle tissue, instead dying off in a matter of days.

Scientists have discovered that the aging process doesn't just deplete muscle stem cells, it disrupts the supportive environment, or "niche," that helps them function. Just as a plant requires particular growing conditions — a certain kind of soil, a specific amount of water, and the right amount of sunlight — so do these stem cells. Without the right molecular signals, transplanted stem cells simply cannot "take root."

To get around this issue, researchers are starting to develop ways to "prime" stem-cell niches prior to transplantation — that way, any new muscle stem cells we inject will have the best chance of surviving. This practice is already commonplace in bone marrow transplants, where researchers usually remove all of the remaining bone marrow before inserting any new marrow. With the old cells removed, the new cells don't need to fight for a place in the tissue

— they can settle wherever they see fit. Similarly, eradication of existing muscle stem cells before transplantation has boosted the survival rate of the new muscle stem cells. Transplanted stem cells seem to "prefer" being able to carve out their own niche instead of settling into old niches.

In fact, priming stem-cell niches in this way has led to a massive leap in our ability to keep transplanted stem cells alive: usually, such stem cells die a few days after being introduced and fail to properly integrate with the muscle tissue. But with the primed microenvironment, we've now been able to keep muscle stem cells surviving for upwards of four months. And crucially, these transplanted stem cells are able to help regenerate damaged muscle tissue following a series of different injuries, proving that they fully integrate into the niche.

Like with the heart stem cells I discussed in the last chapter, muscle stem cells can also benefit from specialized scaffolding to support them during their growth. These are engineered structures that mimic the physical and chemical properties of a healthy niche, simultaneously protecting transplanted cells as well as guiding their integration.

## From Lab to Pharmacy?

The fight against sarcopenia is advancing on multiple fronts, with exercise mimetics and stem-cell therapies offering new possibilities to restore and maintain muscle health as we age. But while they're promising, these approaches remain largely confined to the laboratory for now, with critical hurdles like safety, efficacy, and scalability still to be addressed. Bridging the gap between experimental success and practical application will require ongoing research, robust clinical trials, and regulatory frameworks to ensure these therapies are both accessible and equitable. In the meantime, exercise remains the gold standard for preserving muscle mass and strength, a time-tested intervention that continues to set the benchmark for future innovations. So, go lift some heavy things and put them down again — then, rinse and repeat.

~~*

## Osteoporosis: These Old Bones

Muscles are what allow us to move — they're the engines of our body. But, they would be nothing without the scaffolding that supports them: our skeleton. This is what gives our muscles, and us, structure.

Imagine your skeleton as a bustling construction site, constantly under renovation. Every day, specialized teams of workers are busy tearing down old, worn-out sections and building new, stronger ones. This never-ending project is what keeps your bones healthy and strong throughout your life.

The foremen of this skeletal construction crew are two types of cells: osteoblasts are the builders and osteoclasts are the demolition experts. Yet, these cells don't work in isolation; they're in constant communication, sending chemical messages back and forth to coordinate their efforts. Some of these messages, like cytokines and growth factors, are like local radio broadcasts, affecting only nearby cells. Others, such as hormones, are more like national news broadcasts, influencing cells throughout the entire skeleton.

With age, this highly organized construction site starts to fall into chaos. The osteoblast builders slow down, while the osteoclast demolition crews keep working at full speed or even pick up the pace. It's as if the construction site has more wrecking balls than cement mixers. The result? More bone is torn down than rebuilt, leading to weaker, more fragile bones — a condition we call osteoporosis. By learning how to tune into and adjust these cellular conversations, scientists hope to find ways to keep our skeletal construction crews working in harmony well into our golden years.

## Can We Turn Old Bones Young Again?

Bones are special. They are one of the few tissues in the body that can completely regenerate. No scars, no blemishes — as good as new. The unsung heroes in charge of this feat are called skeletal stem and progenitor cells (SSPCs). They reside in the bone marrow, where they help keep things in balance and can be called upon to replace old or damaged bone cells. These skeletal stem cells can differentiate into two distinct cell types: osteoblasts, which help secrete the scaffolding for bone formation, or adipocytes, which are fat cells that act as stores of energy within the skeletal niche. Between the two, our bones are kept in shape and ready to carry us through life.

Unfortunately, the delicate balance between these two cell types is interrupted as we age. Stem cells begin to develop a bias, preferentially developing into fat cells over their bone-forming counterparts. This leads to a decline in mineral density within the bone marrow and an increase in fat content. To make things worse, adipose cells actively release signals that curb the production and regeneration of bone. We are left with "imbalanced" bones that are significantly more fragile and vulnerable to harm.

Scientists are now uncovering the secrets behind this shift, and all arrows pointing towards a signaling pathway called "Notch." Picture this pathway as a series of traffic lights that guide skeletal stem cells, determining whether they turn into osteoblasts (bone builders) or adipocytes (fat-storing cells). During embryonic development, Notch signaling is crucial for shaping the skeleton, which initially forms as cartilage before gradually turning into bone. At this stage, Notch operates at full intensity, ensuring proper skeletal formation and cellular decision-making.

Yet this pathway begins to malfunction as we get older — a story you know all too well at this point. Instead of efficiently directing traffic, it behaves like a traffic light stuck on green, only allowing some cars through while others are left waiting at the red light. The consequence? An increasing bias toward the formation of fat cells at the expense of bone-building cells.

By restoring balance to this "traffic light" in experimental models, researchers have shown they can reinvigorate aged stem cells, sparking a resurgence in the formation of strong, "fat-free" bones. Essentially, by fixing the traffic light we can tell our stem cells to keep developing into osteoblasts instead of adipocytes.

These breakthroughs not only deepen our understanding of age-related bone degeneration but also lay the groundwork for innovative therapies. We might one day be able to develop drugs that guide aging stem cells back onto the path of bone regeneration, offering new hope for reversing the effects of osteoporosis. And while these remain out of our grasp for now — safety and efficacy still needs to be tested in humans — it's only a matter of time.

## microRNAs: Small Molecules, Big Impact

Although almost all of our cells contain the same DNA, many perform vastly different functions. How? Our genes can be turned "on" or "off". This is known as gene regulation, and determines which set of instructions — or genes — will actually be "expressed". Different genes create different proteins, and thus shape the state and function of a cell. For example, your liver cells don't need to send neurotransmitters, so they keep that gene "turned off". Neurons, on the other hand, *do* rely on neurotransmitters to send signals, so they express the relevant genes.

MicroRNAs are one mechanism by which gene expression is regulated; DNA methylation, as you'll recall from the chapter on epigenetic clocks, is another. But rather than intervening at the root — blocking or activating genes — microRNAs instead intervene at the protein-production stage. These tiny slivers of RNA attach themselves to larger sequences called messenger RNA (mRNA), which provide the genetic information used as a blueprint for the production of proteins. Once attached, the microRNA either cuts out the section of messenger RNA that encodes the target protein, or it just sits on top of the messenger RNA, blocking it from being turned into a protein. Either way, a certain protein that would otherwise have been made is instead suppressed. The outcome is the same as "turning off" the gene itself.

One particular microRNA, dubbed microRNA-141-3p, has emerged as a key player in age-related bone degeneration. Imagine a factory running smoothly thanks to a diligent operations manager —a protein called AUF1— who ensures the machinery works efficiently, keeps defective parts from clogging the system, and prevents dangerous malfunctions. Now imagine that a saboteur sneaks into the control room. This saboteur, microRNA-141-3p, quietly disables the operations manager's ability to oversee the factory. As the saboteur gains influence, chaos ensues: defective machinery piles up, harmful outputs increase, and the entire system begins to break down.

In the context of your cells, this is exactly what happens as microRNA-141-3p levels rise with age. AUF1's ability to stabilize genetic messages and prevent inflammation is compromised, leading to the buildup of inflammatory signals and senescent cells. Over time, this cellular chaos contributes to weakening bones and muscles.

Scientists are now working on strategies to disarm this saboteur. By using molecules called antagomirs to block microRNA-141-3p, they aim to restore AUF1's control over the system. Early studies in animals show promising results: elderly mice, equivalent to humans in their 60s, injected with an antagomir targeting microRNA-141-3p over the course of three months showed reduced inflammation, denser bones, and healthier muscle fibers compared to untreated mice. These changes collectively rejuvenated the tissues, making them appear far younger under a microscope.

As is to be expected, it might be a while until this approach is deemed safe for human use; but, if nothing else, it represents an exciting avenue for the treatment of age-related bone damage.

## Newly Discovered Cells May Help Against Osteoarthritis

Osteoarthritis has long been considered a "wear-and-tear" disease — with repeated movement and a lifetime of activity, the cartilage and other connective tissues in our joints begin to erode. Unsurprisingly, age is a primary risk factor for osteoarthritis. The problem? The exact cause of the disease is unknown, meaning all currently available treatments are just bandages on a broken leg; they help to manage symptoms but fail to reverse the loss of cartilage.

## Secret Progenitor Cells?

In 2019, half a billion people across the globe were living with osteoarthritis — a 113% increase from 1990. It primarily affects the elderly, with 10% of people over the age of 60 suffering from the condition, often forcing significant lifestyle changes and a decrease in physical activity. The inability to move freely can restrict people's ability to engage and participate in meaningful activities, leading to psychological stress and discontent. Osteoarthritis is also frequently accompanied by severe pain, and stiffening of the affected joints is not uncommon. And since we don't really have any long-term treatment options available to us, one in 10 patients will eventually require joint-replacement surgery, an invasive and costly procedure.

While it is understood that osteoarthritis is a result of cartilage loss, which leaves the bones underneath unprotected and exposed to mechanical stress, it is unclear why cartilage is lost in the first place. The "wear-and-tear" explanation suggests that it is simply a result of accumulated strain over years of joint use. In a sense, it's a repetitive-movement injury. But at a biological level, something must be driving the loss of cartilage.

With this as a guiding thread, scientists have recently managed to unearth a previously unknown subset of cartilage progenitor cells defined by the presence of a gene called *Gremlin 1 (grem1)*. Progenitor cells are like the understudies of the cellular world — waiting in the wings, ready to step in and perform specific tasks when needed. While they aren't as versatile as stem cells, which can become almost any type of cell in the body, progenitor cells are more focused. They are precursors to specific cell types, such as muscle cells or bone cells, and play a crucial role in repair and regeneration. Cartilage progenitor cells, for example, "sit" on the articular surfaces of joints — where the bones meet — and develop into cartilage and bone to help fortify the joints as needed.

Notably, mice suffering from osteoarthritis have far fewer of these newly discovered cells than their healthy counterparts. Indeed, genetic removal of the cells quickly leads to the development of osteoarthritis. And in normal mice suffering from osteoarthritis, the progenitor cells are lost during the earliest stages of disease onset.

But with knowledge comes possibility: now that we have a better sense of the core mechanisms that lead to osteoarthritis, we can start finding ways to cure the disease (instead of just treating its symptoms). Already, we're uncovering some promising candidates: mice treated with a protein called fibroblast growth factor 18 (FGF18) — which is part of a larger family of proteins intimately involved in cell survival and tissue repair — enjoyed a stark uptick in the number of *grem1* progenitor cells present in their joint cartilage. This uptick in progenitor cells was accompanied by significant recovery of the joints, including improved cartilage thickness and reduced osteoarthritis.

Unlike some of the other approaches mentioned in this chapter, this one may soon bear fruit. In 2021, findings from a five-year clinical trial were released regarding the use of fibroblast growth factor 18, also known as Sprifermin. The study revealed solid long-term clinical advantages and raised no safety concerns. The drug is currently being tested in a phase III clinical trial. Whereas phases I and II of a trial test specifically for efficacy and safety, phase III tests a drug's performance against the leading available treatment option. It is the last stage of testing before a drug can be approved for use on the market.

## Working Smarter: Drug Repurposing for Osteoarthritis

Developing new drugs is a formidable challenge. It often takes years — if not decades — and costs billions to bring a novel therapeutic to market. For diseases like osteoarthritis, where effective treatments are still hard to come by, this process can feel frustratingly slow. That's where drug repurposing steps in. This approach focuses on finding new uses for drugs that are already approved for other conditions. By skipping many of the early development hurdles, repurposing can save time, resources, and even lives.

Advanced computational tools, including artificial intelligence (AI), have revolutionized drug repurposing. Using vast databases of biomedical data, AI models can identify hidden connections between drugs and diseases, suggesting novel therapeutic applications. For instance, Graph Neural Networks (GNNs) excel at analyzing complex relationships in biomedical data, such as mapping how drugs interact with genetic pathways associated with specific conditions. This approach has become a cornerstone in modern repurposing strategies, enabling scientists to sift through mountains of data and uncover unexpected therapeutic opportunities for osteoarthritis (and beyond).

## Sodium Channels Damage Joints?

Recent discoveries have spotlighted Nav1.7, a sodium channel previously thought to function exclusively in neurons, as a critical factor in osteoarthritis. While traditionally associated with transmitting pain signals, Nav1.7 has now been found in chondrocytes — some of the cells responsible for maintaining healthy cartilage.

Here's the remarkable part: although Nav1.7 channels are sparse in chondrocytes, their impact is immense. In particular, they regulate the delicate processes of building up cartilage (anabolism) and breaking it down (catabolism). When these go haywire, as is often the case in older age, they skew the balance towards breakdown.

Blocking these sodium channels in mouse models — either genetically or through drugs — has thus been linked to significantly reduced cartilage damage, less inflammation, and improved joint mobility. This discovery has opened the door to exploring drugs that block Nav1.7, such as carbamazepine (a drug already used to treat epilepsy), as potential disease-modifying treatments for osteoarthritis.

Of course, there are challenges (there always are): Nav1.7 inhibitors designed for nerve cells may not work as effectively in cartilage. This means researchers will need to tweak available drugs to ensure they target chondrocytes without causing side effects. Additionally, while studies in mice have been promising, human joints are more complex. Large-scale clinical trials are needed to determine whether these treatments can deliver on their promise.

# CHAPTER 26

# The Aging Brain: Challenges and Breakthroughs in Cognitive Longevity

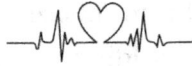

C ognitive decline is one of the most daunting challenges of aging. Though there are multiple facets to cognitive aging, one of its most distressing effects is on our memory, which begins to fade until, in worst-case scenarios, we are left unable to remember who we are.

Since the time of Aristotle and Plato — and realistically, long before — we humans have concerned ourselves with personal identity: What makes *me* who I am? What separates me from you? And, perhaps a more extreme version, what connects the 'me' of today to the 'me' of a decade ago? What is it that allows there to be a cohesive sense of self spanning these chunks of time? One pretty convincing answer to these questions is the "memory-theory of identity." This theory suggests that our sense of self is fundamentally tied to our memories. It posits that who we are — our identity — is shaped by the continuity of experiences, emotions, and thoughts that we can recall and connect over time.

When cognitive decline sets in, it doesn't just erode memory; it disrupts this continuity, creating fractures in the narrative we hold about ourselves. For many, this loss of memory translates to a loss of self, as familiar faces, cherished experiences, and even deeply ingrained habits slip out of reach. This profound threat to identity is one reason cognitive aging strikes such a deep emotional chord

— it's not just about forgetting, but about losing the threads that make us who we are.

Today, nearly one in three people who reach 65 will face severe cognitive impairment or dementia at some point in their lives. As our population grows older, these numbers are set to skyrocket. By 2060, over 15 million Americans are projected to experience moderate to severe cognitive impairment — a figure that carries immense personal and societal costs.

A major reason for the lack of established treatments lies in the immense complexity of the brain itself. Unlike most other organs, the brain's inner workings are still not fully understood, leaving many mechanisms of age-related dementia — and conditions like Alzheimer's disease — shrouded in mystery. This uncertainty has made it difficult to develop reliable interventions, forcing researchers to grapple with the unknown as they strive for solutions.

This means that a significant step in developing therapies for cognitive decline lies in better understanding the condition itself. As we learn to identify the early warning signs and learn to pinpoint where interventions can have the greatest impact, we can refine our focus, turning vast unknowns into actionable insights.

~~

## Klotho: "Miracle Molecule"?

The story of klotho begins with a serendipitous discovery in the 1990s that has since transformed our understanding of aging at a molecular level. The protein was first identified in a lab where researchers were studying high blood pressure in mice. A genetic accident in one of their experiments silenced an unknown gene, resulting in mice that aged at an accelerated pace. These mice developed brittle bones, calcified arteries, and all died prematurely. Intrigued, the scientists named the affected gene "klotho" and embarked on a journey to uncover its secrets.

The name refers to the Greek mythological story of the three Fates. Klotho spun the thread of human life. The two other fates, Lachesis and Atropos, dispensed and cut the thread. Together, the three fates controlled the lives of each human being and had the power to choose who was saved and who passed away. An apt name, albeit slightly dramatic, for the newly discovered protein!

The initial discovery led to another striking revelation: boosting klotho levels in mice not only delayed the onset of age-related diseases but also extended their lifespan. Humans, it turned out, also possess a *klotho* gene, 85% identical to its mouse counterpart. The protein exists in several forms, acting both locally in tissues like the kidney and brain and systemically, akin to a hormone. Its effects are far-reaching, influencing everything from kidney and cardiovascular health to brain function and bone strength.

One of the primary ways that klotho is suspected to increase longevity is by acting as an anti-inflammatory protein. Inflammation is part of the body's defense against harmful stimuli such as viruses or damaged cells. Controlled inflammatory responses are necessary for protecting our bodies and keeping us healthy. But when inflammatory responses are uncontrolled or chronic, they can hurt the body more than they help (just think back to the chapter on chronic inflammation).

A number of experiments have now shown that klotho inhibits two key players in the inflammation process. One of these is NF-kB, which is a transcription factor critical for the activation of the entire inflammatory pathway. Transcription factors regulate the production of proteins from genes in the body. NF-kB, specifically, plays a crucial role in regulating the production of inflammatory proteins.

The second is tumor necrosis factor-alpha (TNF-alpha). TNF-alpha is a cytokine and is also a major regulator of the inflammatory response. Cytokines act as messengers and send signals to other immune cells, recruiting them to areas of injury.

## Klotho and Brain Health

Chronic inflammation in the brain has been linked to several diseases including Alzheimer's disease and brain fog. With its anti-inflammatory properties, there is suspicion that the klotho protein may play a role in protecting the brain against inflammatory neurological diseases and neurodegenerative diseases. A version of the protein, named "alpha-klotho," is highly abundant in a central structure of the brain called the choroid plexus. The choroid plexus is a network of blood vessels that produce cerebrospinal fluid, which is vital for providing the brain with nutrients and protection. Recent studies on "cultured cells" — a term for cells that have been grown in a lab dish — have confirmed as much; introduction of alpha-klotho significantly reduces markers of inflammation.

Beyond cutting down inflammation, klotho also appears to actively protect our brain cells. Neurodegenerative disorders like Alzheimer's and Parkinson's disease are defined by the progressive death of our neuronal brain cells. In experiments, lab-grown neurons that are pre-treated with alpha-klotho have a much higher chance of surviving in the face of inflammation. That said, it is only protective up to a point — when exposed to higher levels of inflammation, there was no difference in neuronal death compared to the control group (those neurons that did not receive the alpha-klotho pre-treatment).

While we are still figuring out *how* klotho works — the ins and outs of the mechanisms — we do know *that* it works. Our bodies naturally produce Klotho in the kidneys in two forms: a protein that inserts itself into cell membranes and a secreted hormone that circulates the bloodstream. As we age, levels of the hormone version naturally decline. Emerging mouse studies, however, have found that injecting klotho directly into the bloodstream preserves memory and even reverses age-related cognitive decline. Although klotho does not seem to cross the blood-brain barrier — a protective "bubble" around the brain in charge of deciding what is allowed to enter and exit — introducing low doses of the hormone into mice has been shown to boost working memory and increase neural plasticity. Indeed, their brains undergo significant changes that allow more connections to be made in the hippocampus, the brain's learning and memory center.

## Not Just Mice, Monkeys Too

But mice aren't humans. They aren't even primates. So, how seriously can we take these results? Well, more recent follow-up studies have confirmed that the same boost in thinking and memory can be replicated in older monkeys. These, whether we like it or not, are genetically very similar to us — primate studies are generally a better predictor of human outcomes than studies based on mice. Of course, neither is really a perfect stand-in for human studies, but we need to start somewhere (especially when we don't yet have a good sense of possible side effects and risks).

The team from Yale University began their experiments by synthesizing a hormone form of klotho that is naturally produced by monkeys. They then administered a dose of klotho, via injection, to a group of adult monkeys. These monkeys, in "human years," ranged from 45 to 85 years of age, allowing investigators to determine whether klotho can reverse age-related cognitive decline.

The experiments were completed over the course of three months. In the first month, the monkeys learned to complete spatial delayed-response tasks that measured normal and high memory load. The normal memory load task was simple. Each monkey was presented with four wells, one of which contained a cue for a food reward. After a few moments, a screen dropped down to obscure their view of the wells. Once the wall came up, the monkey was able to retrieve the food reward by reaching into the well that had contained the cue. To test high memory load, the investigators increased the number of wells, as well as the time between the cue and testing phase. Their performance from these tasks were used to measure their baseline cognitive function.

After this first set of experiments, all the monkeys underwent a scam injection to habituate them to stress of the procedure. In the days following the sham injection, they underwent another round of normal and high memory load tasks. Investigators did not observe a difference in performance compared to the initial baseline scores, confirming that the injection process itself had no impact on cognition.

Finally, a group of monkeys were injected with the synthesized klotho hormone. As expected, they performed far better on both the normal and high memory load tasks. The treated monkeys continued to outperform the control group for more than two weeks after the klotho had been given. Excitingly, the benefits of klotho were not only immediate (within four hours of the injection) but also long-lasting, suggesting that this hormone may enhance long-term memory.

While still early, these results are extremely promising and suggest that, with a bit more research, we might soon be able to exploit the protective powers of klotho for therapeutic use. In the same way you go to your doctor for yearly flu vaccinations, you may soon be able to go in for a yearly klotho boost to help your brain keep doing what it does best: think, remember, and find meaning.

~⁓

## Platelet Factor-4 (PF4): One to Watch

What do blood transfusions, exercise, and a longevity hormone have in common? All three help improve cognitive health and, to varying extents, rejuvenate the brain. But until recently, no one could pinpoint the specific molecule responsible for the improvements. That's now changing, with researchers having cracked the code by tracing the brain-boosting effects of the interventions to a protein called platelet factor-4 (PF4).

## Young Blood, Young Brain

The first study implicating this protein focused on blood transfusions. A team of researchers based at the University of San

Francisco injected old mice with the blood of young mice. They noticed that the influx of young blood brought with it all kinds of health improvements, including stronger muscles and decreased brain inflammation. Somehow, blood from young mice was helping old mice turn back their biological clocks.

By analyzing the blood of the young mice, the scientists discovered that it contained noticeably higher levels of platelet factor-4 than did the blood of old mice. They saw the same thing when comparing the blood of young humans to that of older humans.

To test whether they had stumbled upon the culprit, they isolated platelet factor-4 and injected it directly into old mice, without the addition of any young blood. As before, the old mice began to rejuvenate; inflammation in the brain region linked to memory decreased, brain connectivity increased, and thinking skills improved.

Saul A. Villeda, PhD, senior author of the study, remarked that, "We're taking 22-month-old mice, equivalent to a human in their 70s, and PF4 is bringing them back to function close to their late 30s, early 40s."

## The Benefits of Exercise Without Moving?

You'll remember from our earlier discussion on cardiovascular health that scientists are busy developing ways of "bottling" the benefits of exercise. The heart isn't the only organ that stands to gain from this. The same approach, in fact, may help stave off the cognitive decline we so often see encroaching with age.

Building on a mountain of evidence that exercise helps delay and soften the onset of cognitive decline, a group of Australian scientists sought to isolate the source of these benefits. In earlier work released in 2019, the lab discerned that exercise activates and releases platelets into the bloodstream. These platelets, in turn, activated a number of proteins and hormones, including platelet factor-4. At the time, they tested platelet factor-4 for its ability to stimulate the production of new neurons in the brain, known as neurogenesis. Direct delivery of platelet factor 4 into the brains of mice did manage to enhance neurogenesis, improving memory and slowing age-related cognitive decline.

Spurred on by this initial success, the researchers returned to confirm whether the same effects could be achieved through systemic delivery of platelet facto- 4 — through the bloodstream, which, as you can imagine, is much less invasive than direct delivery into the brain. As expected, old mice again showed increases in neurogenesis and a general restoration of cognitive function.

## An Old Friend: Klotho

While talking about klotho, I mentioned something strange: when injected into the bloodstream, the protein doesn't appear to be able to travel through the blood-brain barrier. Yet, despite this, it clearly manages to impact various brain regions, including the hippocampus. How? There has to be some kind of middleman at play. If klotho isn't crossing the barrier, it must be activating some other molecule that does.

We now have an answer to this riddle thanks to a team based at the University of California, San Francisco. After injecting mice with klotho, the scientists noticed a sharp spike in platelets, and subsequently, various proteins released by these platelets. One of these was none other than platelet factor-4 (PF4). To make sure they were on the right track, the team blocked the platelet response to see what would happen. As expected, blocking the platelets also blocked the cognitive benefits usually associated with klotho — the platelets were necessary for klotho to be able to have its positive effects.

The researchers next homed in on platelet factor-4, quickly verifying that injection of the protein by itself was enough to trigger the same improvements to cognition and memory seen during injection with klotho. But one important thing to note is that mice engineered to be lacking platelet factor-4 still benefited from klotho, suggesting that other platelet factors may also play a role in the klotho's healing abilities. Future work should aim to identify these other platelet factors and help fill in the gaps in our understanding.

## Risk of Blood Clots

Although this trifecta of studies is very exciting, we shouldn't get ahead of ourselves. Platelet factor-4 is a natural blood coagulant — it thickens blood to help clog up wounds and stop bleeding at sites of injury. It is a critical component of tissue repair. Although this doesn't sound like a bad thing, it does mean that boosting platelet factor-4 could lead to blood clotting outside of injury contexts. Clotting inside veins and arteries can pose serious risks, including heart attacks or strokes. Before being used therapeutically in humans, any intervention based on platelet factor-4 would need rigorous safety testing to make sure it does not increase the risk of harmful blood clots. Potential risks aside, emerging research makes a compelling case for the importance of platelet factor-4 in cognitive health, including critical thinking and memory. And the study involving klotho also indicates that there may be other, as-yet-unknown platelet factors that hold similar roles.

~~

## Light And Sound Therapy to Treat Cognitive Decline?

Alzheimer's is a notoriously tricky condition; despite throwing a great deal of effort, and resources, towards understanding it, there are still more unknowns than knowns. This is most apparent when considering the relative lack of treatment options. For a life-altering disease that impacts so many people, it's shocking how few effective interventions we have. And those that are available, like Leqembi, are often cost-prohibitive, with an annual price tag in the tens of thousands.

With this in mind, you may be surprised to hear that a fairly simple and non-invasive approach has been yielding promising results: stimulating the brain with 40-hertz frequencies, whether light or sound. This has proved an exciting new avenue for treatment, with a handful of successful early trials.

Let's back up for a moment: why did anyone think to use flashing lights to treat Alzheimer's in the first place? To answer this, we need to take a quick detour through some basic neuroscience.

Brain functions are regulated by the communication of a synchronized network of brain cells called neurons. These send signals to one another, and across the nervous system, by way of electrical impulses. Neuronal activity of this kind follows certain patterns or rhythms, more commonly known as "brain waves". When you get an electroencephalography (EEG), for example, doctors are essentially looking at the rhythm of your brain's tides.

Well, gamma waves — characterized by an oscillation pattern of 40 cycles, or hertz, per second — are some of the fastest brain waves, intimately linked to the connectivity of different brain regions. They are thought to play an active role in both memory and sustained attention.

Back in 2016, a group of researchers at the Massachusetts Institute of Technology (MIT) led by Dr. Li-Huei Tsai noticed that gamma waves were unusually inactive in mice suffering from Alzheimer's disease. This was particularly noticeable in the hippocampus. The results piqued their interest; would artificially boosting gamma-wave activity help fight off cognitive decline? A few experiments later, they concluded that exposing mice to a light flickering at 40 hertz did, in fact, help cut down amyloid plaques, a hallmark of Alzheimer's, by almost 50%.

Since then, the Tsai Laboratory has gone on to perform numerous follow-up studies, all of which indicate that lights flashing at 40 cycles per second, or sounds clicking at the same frequency, can reduce the symptoms of Alzheimer's disease in mice. Two early-stage human studies helped confirm the safety of the approach and suggest that the benefits seen in mice may also be available to us.

But through all this, one thing remained frustratingly unclear: how, and why, does gamma stimulation stave off cognitive decline? What are the mechanisms at the biological and molecular levels?

## The Brain's Very Own Plumbing System

The latest round of experiments by the Tsai Laboratory has offered some insight: the findings suggest that 40-hertz stimulation works by boosting a recently discovered "plumbing system" in the brain, called the glymphatic system, which flushes out metabolic waste, including the infamous amyloid plaques associated with Alzheimer's disease.

Our body is constantly producing waste products — substances that are left over from metabolic processes, such as protein synthesis, but cannot be put to any other use. If these waste products are left to pile up, they begin to have toxic effects on the surrounding tissues. Not good.

In most regions of the body, the responsibility for preventing this kind of clogging falls on the lymphatic system. This system is made up of a large network of "pipes", called lymph vessels, filled with a fluid called lymph. Cells excrete waste products into interstitial fluid, which surrounds and separates cells. This fluid, filled with all the cellular "sewage", moves into the lymph vessels, where it merges with the lymph and is carried away to be filtered, broken down, and eventually removed — think urination, or well, the other one.

But the central nervous system, despite being an especially sensitive system, does not contain any lymphatic structures. Still, it is somehow very efficient at clearing waste. This left researchers scratching their heads. If the lymphatic system doesn't extend to the brain, how are waste products and debris being removed? In 2012, a group of Danish scientists discovered what they dubbed the "glymphatic" system. Basically, the brain's very own, custom-made lymphatic system.

The glymphatic system is made of tiny, specialized channels that follow along the blood vessels of the brain, giving cerebrospinal fluid — a colorless fluid that surrounds the brain and provides nutrients — quick and easy access to all areas. Think of pipes in a house transporting water to wherever it's needed. Traveling along these channels, cerebrospinal fluid is flushed into the "meaty" tissue of the brain, where it mixes with soiled interstitial fluid. The cerebrospinal fluid picks up all of the waste products in the spaces between neurons before being flushed out again through the same channels, leaving behind clean interstitial fluid. The waste products are then sent to the lymph nodes in the neck for filtering and disposal.

## How Gamma Waves Protect The Brain

To test whether 40-hertz stimulation influences the glymphatic system, Tsai and her colleagues checked if the intervention was linked to any changes in the flow of fluids in the brain. They found that mice treated with gamma stimulation had more cerebrospinal fluid in their brain tissue compared to untreated mice. They also noticed that the fluid left the brain more quickly in the treated mice, possibly due to a physical enlargement of the special glymphatic channels. Finally, the lymph nodes in the necks of the mice that received 40-hertz stimulation were full of amyloid beta compared to those of the control group, suggesting that the harmful protein had successfully been drained out of the brain.

One likely explanation for these changes can be traced to a protein called aquaporin 4. This is a water-channel protein, meaning it helps direct fluids through cell membranes. The "feet" of astrocytes, a special kind of brain cell, are covered with aquaporin 4, allowing them to mediate glymphatic fluid exchange. Blocking the protein, either chemically or genetically, also blocks the benefits of the 40-hertz brain stimulation, indicating that it plays a crucial role in the benefits associated with the treatment.

Another potential explanation for the effectiveness of 40-hertz stimulation is the discovery that interneurons — a subset of neurons — produce certain peptides in far greater quantities following treatment. This includes a peptide known as vasoactive intestinal polypeptide (VIP), which is understood to have Alzehimer's-busting effects and is associated with the regulation of blood flow and glymphatic clearance. As with aquaporin 4, blocking the expression of vasoactive intestinal polypeptide also blocked the clearance of amyloid beta; the effectiveness of the gamma stimulation fell apart.

So, gamma-wave treatment improves the efficacy of the brain's waste-management system. This, in turn, helps clear up accumulated debris and proteins which, if left unattended, would cause damage. With ongoing trials aimed at converting these lab results into practical applications — wearable glasses that stimulate the brain with 40-hertz lights — we may soon have a non-invasive and affordable treatment option for early-stage Alzheimer's disease. Compared to our current options, which can be counted on one hand, this would represent a massive leap forward.

# CHAPTER 27

# Cancer: The Great Scourge of Aging

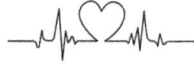

C ancer. The word alone has a way of stopping us in our tracks, conjuring an image of one of our most formidable foes. Despite decades of research and remarkable advances, cancer remains a leading cause of mortality worldwide, claiming millions of lives each year. It's a disease that touches almost everyone in some way — whether through a personal diagnosis, a loved one's battle, or a constant reminder of its pervasiveness in society.

Cancer cells are, in a sense, the ultimate survivors. They harness the very mechanisms that keep healthy cells alive — growth, adaptation, and repair — but twist them into weapons of unchecked proliferation. Like rebels in an otherwise orderly society, they evade the body's systems of checks and balances, hijacking resources to fuel their relentless expansion. Yet, for all their cunning, cancer cells also expose vulnerabilities that the medical sciences are learning to exploit.

Today, the arsenal against cancer is more sophisticated than ever. Beyond the familiar pillars of surgery, radiation, and chemotherapy, modern medicine is exploring targeted therapies that precisely strike cancer cells while sparing healthy tissue. Immunotherapy, which trains the body's immune system to recognize and destroy cancer, is transforming outcomes for certain types of the disease. Even experimental approaches, like genetically engineered viruses and nanotechnology, are making headlines for their potential to revolutionize treatment. From therapies that turn the body's defenses into allies to innovations that seek to prevent cancer altogether, this chapter is a journey into one of the most dynamic frontiers of modern medicine.

~●

## What is it? What Causes it?

Cancer is not a foreign invader. It doesn't come from outside the body, like an infection or toxin. Instead, it arises from within, a betrayal of the very cells that make up our bodies. At its core, cancer is a breakdown of cellular discipline. Normal cells follow a set of instructions — when to divide, when to repair, and when to die for the greater good. Cancer cells, however, abandon these rules. They begin to multiply uncontrollably, refusing to die on schedule, forming masses that disrupt the body's balance.

Why does this happen? The causes of cancer are as varied as the disease itself. Sometimes, the trigger is external — exposure to harmful substances like tobacco, ultraviolet radiation, or certain chemicals. These kinds of external triggers are called "carcinogens."Other times, the problem begins at the genetic level. Mutations, or errors in our DNA, can accumulate over time, disabling the very mechanisms that keep cell growth in check. These mutations may be inherited, but often they are acquired throughout life as our cells divide and interact with the environment.

Broadly speaking, cancers fall into two major categories. Some arise in the blood, where they disrupt the normal production of vital cells like red and white blood cells. These are known as blood cancers, such as leukemia, lymphoma, or myeloma, and they often originate in the bone marrow or immune system. In contrast, solid tumors form masses of tissue in organs like the lungs, breasts, or colon. While blood cancers spread through the circulatory system, solid tumors can grow locally or metastasize — the medical term for "move" — to other parts of the body. These two categories behave differently, requiring distinct approaches to treatment and presenting unique challenges for researchers and clinicians alike.

Among the many risk factors for cancer, one stands out above all others: age. As we grow older, our cells have more opportunities to accumulate damage. Think of DNA as a manuscript of instructions. Over decades of editing and re-editing, typos inevitably slip through the cracks, disrupting the flow and meaning of the text. These "typos" in our DNA can lead to the unregulated growth that defines cancer. It's no surprise, then, that cancer is overwhelmingly a disease of aging; nearly 80% of cancer diagnoses occur in people over 55.

But age isn't the only factor. Lifestyle choices, like smoking or diet, play a significant role, as does prolonged exposure to carcinogens, chronic inflammation, and even certain viruses. Genetics can also predispose some individuals to cancer, meaning they start the race with fewer protective mechanisms in place. It's this interplay — between environment, genetics, and the passage of time — that makes cancer so challenging to prevent and treat.

## CAR-T Cell Therapy: Reprogramming the Immune System to Fight Cancer

The immune system is nature's vigilant guardian, always on the lookout for harmful invaders. But cancer, with its uncanny ability to masquerade as normal tissue, often evades detection, growing unchecked. CAR-T cell therapy changes that, transforming regular immune cells into specialized warriors with a singular mission: to seek out and destroy cancer.

CAR-T cell therapy, short for chimeric antigen receptor T-cell therapy, begins with a patient's own immune cells. Specifically, T cells — immune cells responsible for identifying and attacking threats — are harvested from the bloodstream. In the lab, these cells undergo genetic engineering to express chimeric antigen receptors (CARs) on their surface. These receptors act like homing devices, enabling the T cells to recognize specific proteins, or antigens, found on the surface of cancer cells. Once modified, the CAR-T cells are multiplied in large numbers and infused back into the patient, where they begin their mission of tracking down and eliminating cancer cells.

## History of CAR-T Therapy

The journey to CAR-T therapy's success has been anything but straightforward. The concept of using the immune system to combat cancer dates back to the early 20th century, but it wasn't until the 1990s that the idea of genetically modifying T cells began to take shape. Early attempts faced significant obstacles. The first-generation CARs were rudimentary, leading to poor persistence and lackluster results.

But advances in genetic engineering and a deeper understanding of T-cell biology allowed for the development of second- and third-generation CARs, which were designed to be more effective and longer-lasting. These improvements included the addition of "signaling domains" — specific molecular components within the engineered T cells that boost their ability to attack cancer cells. Think of these signaling domains as built-in amplifiers that hone the T cells' response once they detect a cancer cell. With these enhancements, the modified T cells can stay active for longer periods and mount a more aggressive attack, significantly improving their ability to fight off cancer.

Then, in 2017, we hit a clear milestone: the U.S. Food and Drug Administration (FDA) approved the first CAR-T therapy for acute lymphoblastic leukemia (ALL) in children and young adults. Acute lymphoblastic leukemia is a fast-growing cancer of the blood and bone marrow where immature white blood cells multiply uncontrollably, crowding out healthy cells. For patients who had exhausted traditional options like chemotherapy or radiation, CAR-T therapy provided a groundbreaking alternative. Shortly after, this therapy was also approved for certain types of lymphoma, another category of blood cancers that affect the lymphatic system, part of the body's immune defenses.

These approvals marked a transformative moment in cancer treatment. CAR-T therapy demonstrated that it could succeed where conventional approaches had failed, offering hope to patients who once faced limited options.

## How Well Does it Work?

CAR-T cell therapy's impact lies in its ability to deliver extraordinary outcomes, particularly for patients with the most challenging cases of cancer. These include relapsed cancers, which have returned after initial treatment, and refractory cancers, which fail to respond to traditional therapies like chemotherapy or radiation. For these patients — who often face grim prognoses — CAR-T offers a lifeline.

Clinical trials have reported overall response rates exceeding 80% for some blood cancers. Even more remarkable, many achieved complete remission, where all signs of cancer disappear, and tests show no detectable disease — a result that would have been unthinkable a decade ago.

Critically, unlike many cancer treatments that merely stall progression, CAR-T therapies aim for durable remissions. Patients who achieve complete remission often enjoy long-term survival without relapse, a distinction that sets CAR-T apart from traditional options like chemotherapy and radiation. In some cases, these therapies have even demonstrated curative potential, inspiring researchers to explore how this success could be replicated across other cancer types.

## What About Solid Tumors?

Remember, cancers fall into two main buckets: those that form in the bloodstream and those that form as solid tumors. While CAR-T therapy has proven remarkably effective against the former, it tends to run into difficulties when faced with solid tumors.

Blood cancers are relatively accessible to T cells circulating in the bloodstream, but solid tumors present a more hostile environment. These tumors are surrounded by dense tissue that acts like a physical barrier, making it harder for immune cells to reach them. Additionally, the proteins on the surface of cancer cells, which CAR-T cells use to identify their targets, often vary widely within a single tumor. This diversity makes it difficult for CAR-T cells to recognize and attack all the cancer cells effectively.

To tackle these obstacles, researchers are exploring various new strategies. One promising development involves "armored CAR-T cells," which are engineered to secrete cytokines — molecules that enhance immune activity — directly into the tumor microenvironment. This effectively kills two birds with one stone: not only do the CAR-T cells eliminate cancer cells but they also transform the hostile tumor environment into one that supports immune activity. For example, CAR-T cells expressing IL-12, a potent cytokine, have shown success in preclinical models by recruiting other immune cells to attack the tumor alongside the CAR-T cells.

We're also making headway by experimenting with different techniques for the administration of CAR-T therapy. Instead of relying on systemic infusion — where the cells circulate throughout the body and struggle to penetrate dense tumor environments — researchers are now opting for direct injections into the tumor itself. This localized approach ensures a higher concentration of CAR-T cells at the tumor site, giving them a better shot at dismantling the cancer. Plus, early trials suggest this method could trigger a domino effect, activating the immune system to attack cancer cells that have spread elsewhere in the body.

While these strategies are still in experimental stages, they may soon make CAR-T therapy a viable option for solid tumors, giving more patients battling hard-to-treat cancers a last line of defense.

## Challenges and Considerations

Despite its promise, CAR-T therapy is not without challenges. For one, there is a risk of side effects. Cytokine release syndrome (CRS), a potentially severe immune reaction, occurs in some patients due to the rapid activation of CAR-T cells. Symptoms range from mild flu-like conditions to life-threatening complications requiring intensive care. Neurotoxicity is another risk — and yes, it's as bad as it sounds. Some patients are left feeling confused, and some suffer seizures or other neurological symptoms. And while these risks are substantial, they underscore the immense power of CAR-T therapy — these are the side effects of an immune system revving up to fight cancer with extreme vigor.

Another challenge facing CAR-T therapy is its cost and complexity, which make it inaccessible to many of those who could most benefit from it. The entire process — from harvesting T cells to engineering them in a lab and then reinfusing them into the patient — is incredibly labor-intensive. Each treatment is customized for the individual, and this personalization comes at a steep price. Here in the United States, a single course of CAR-T therapy can come with a hefty $400,000 price tag, not including hospital stays or follow-up care.

The complexity of the procedure also means it requires highly trained staff and cutting-edge facilities, creating additional barriers to widespread use. For CAR-T therapy to truly live up to its promise of revolutionizing cancer care, these barriers need to be broken down. Whether through innovations that simplify how the therapy is made, advancements in technology to bring down costs, or healthcare policies that ensure broader access, the goal remains the same: making this life-saving treatment a viable option for more people, not just a privileged few.

~~*

## Checkpoint Inhibitors: Releasing the Brakes

Like any well-run security team, the immune system has built-in "brakes" — called immune checkpoints — that prevent it from going overboard and attacking healthy tissue. These brakes are controlled by proteins like PD-1 and CTLA-4, which send "slow down" signals to the immune cells. Such signals are essential for preventing autoimmune diseases, where the immune system becomes overactive and mistakenly attacks the body.

The problem is, cancer cells have learned how to manipulate these checkpoints. By producing proteins like PD-L1 (the partner protein to PD-1), tumors essentially hijack the system, sending out fake "do not attack" signals. This allows cancer to hide in plain sight, growing and spreading while the immune system stands down.

Immune checkpoint inhibitors work by cutting through cancer's camouflage. These drugs target proteins like PD-1, PD-L1, or CTLA-4, which act as the brakes on the immune system. By blocking these proteins, checkpoint inhibitors "release the brakes," allowing T cells to recognize and attack cancer cells. This approach, part of the broader field of immunotherapy, has become a game-changer in treating cancers like melanoma, lung cancer, and Hodgkin lymphoma. Unlike chemotherapy, which directly attacks cancer but can harm healthy tissue in the process, checkpoint inhibitors empower the body's own defenses to do the work, offering a more targeted and often less toxic solution.

## Effectiveness and Impact

Checkpoint inhibitors have produced impressive results for certain cancers. For instance, when it comes to metastatic melanoma — a type of skin cancer that has spread to other parts of the body — checkpoint inhibitors have transformed survival rates, with some patients living years longer than expected. Studies show response rates of up to 40% in advanced cases of melanoma. These therapies have also demonstrated effectiveness in non-small cell lung cancer and kidney cancer, among others, with durable responses in many patients.

But immune checkpoint inhibitors are not a panacea. They work best in cancers that have already triggered a strong immune response, known as "hot" tumors. Cancers with little immune activity, or "cold" tumors, are less responsive.

Additionally, while side effects are generally less severe than chemotherapy, they can still occur. Some patients experience inflammation in healthy organs, like the lungs or liver, as the immune system becomes overzealous. Doctors often use drugs that suppress the immune system, such as corticosteroids, to rein in the immune response. Unfortunately, this approach also blunts the therapy's effectiveness, forcing clinicians to weigh the risks and benefits carefully. What's more, these adverse effects can appear months or even years after treatment, meaning patients require ongoing monitoring long after their initial therapy ends. This has led to a growing emphasis on "survivorship care," ensuring that long-term side effects are recognized and managed effectively.

## Old but Gold: Aging Enhances Checkpoint Inhibitors

There's an unexpected twist to checkpoint inhibitors: age may boost the effectiveness of these therapies. While the immune system generally weakens with age, making older adults more susceptible to infections and slower to heal, checkpoint inhibitors seem to work better in older patients. Why?

At the heart of this phenomenon is the dynamic between two types of immune cells: cytotoxic T cells (the cancer fighters) and regulatory T cells (which keep the immune system in check to prevent overactivation). In younger patients, tumors often contain a higher proportion of regulatory T cells, which suppress the activity of cytotoxic T cells and limit the effectiveness of checkpoint inhibitors. As we age, this balance shifts. Older individuals tend to have fewer regulatory T cells within tumors, allowing cytotoxic T cells to act more freely and making checkpoint inhibitors more effective.

So, while there's still a lot of work to be done, it's reassuring to know that checkpoint inhibitors are most effective when we are most likely to start actually needing them — in old age.

~~

## Prevention is King: A Peek at Cancer Vaccines

Cancer vaccines represent one of the most ambitious goals in oncology: using the body's own immune system to prevent cancer from ever taking root. The concept is deceptively simple: introduce a substance — whether a protein, antigen, or genetic material — that triggers the immune system to recognize and attack cancer cells. Yet, execution of this idea has proven anything but straightforward.

The idea of cancer vaccines isn't new. Research began to ramp up in the early 2000s, leading to notable successes like the FDA-approved HPV vaccine, Gardasil, in 2006. Gardasil has since dramatically reduced rates of cervical and other HPV-related cancers. While preventive vaccines have done well, therapeutic cancer vaccines — designed to treat existing tumors — have been a tougher nut to crack. Sipuleucel-T, approved in 2010, was the first therapeutic cancer vaccine shown to improve survival in patients with advanced prostate cancer, but progress since has been incremental. A string of disappointing late-phase clinical trials over the past decade has forced us to temper much of our initial excitement around cancer vaccines, particularly for therapeutic applications.

That being said, the field is now seeing renewed optimism. Advances in technology — spurred by the success of mRNA vaccines during the COVID-19 pandemic — have reinvigorated research. These can be designed to encode specific tumor antigens, prompting the immune system to mount a targeted attack. The flexibility of this platform allows for rapid customization, making it particularly suited for personalized vaccines, which are tailored to target the unique mutations of an individual's tumor. And they are showing promise in early trials. At the same time, researchers are exploring "off-the-shelf" vaccines that target shared neoantigens, common to many cancers. This dual approach could broaden accessibility while ensuring precision in treatment.

The impact of cancer vaccines, if fully realized, could be transformative. Preventive vaccines like those for HPV have already shown their power, reducing cervical cancer rates dramatically in vaccinated populations. Therapeutic vaccines, while still in their infancy, hold the potential to turn cancer into a manageable condition, akin to how antiretroviral therapies revolutionized HIV care.

With advances in technology and a deeper understanding of tumor biology, cancer vaccines may eventually become a pillar of both prevention and treatment. They remind us that the ultimate goal of cancer research isn't just to cure, but to prevent — a vision of a future where cancer is not a battle to fight, but a threat we've learned to neutralize before it begins.

# Closing Thoughts: How Long is Too Long?

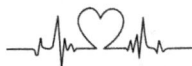

—ᴧᴧᏕ2ᴧᴧᴧ—

Humanity is living longer than ever before. Advances in science, medicine, and public health have extended lifespans to an extraordinary degree. In the early 20th century, life expectancy in many parts of the world hovered around 50 years. Today, it is not uncommon to see people celebrating their 90th birthdays or beyond. This longevity revolution is a triumph of our ingenuity — a testament to what we can achieve when knowledge meets opportunity.

But as we add years to life, we need to remember to pause and ask ourselves: what do these extra years mean? A society where living to 100 becomes the norm will need to rethink fundamental aspects of how we work, educate, and care for one another.

Economically, the challenges are immense. Many pension systems, originally designed for an era where retirement lasted a mere 10 to 15 years, are straining under the weight of an aging population. In countries where public pensions form the backbone of retirement, such as Japan and much of Europe, governments face mounting deficits as payouts increase while the working-age population contributing to these systems dwindles. The resulting pressure is forcing policymakers to reconsider retirement ages, potentially raising them to align with longer life expectancies. You can imagine how that might sit with people — and understandably so. In fact, we've already had a taste of what this may look like: in 2023, over a million people marched and went on strike in France to protest plans to hike up the pension age by two years. While the French people are renowned for their willingness to mobilize and protest, I don't doubt we'll see similar responses around the world.

In the labor market, longer lifespans will likely force us to change how we do things. The traditional model of education, work, and retirement — once considered a linear path — may need to evolve into a more cyclical approach. People might return to education in their 40s or 50s to reskill, take extended career breaks, or engage in phased retirements. Older workers bring decades of experience to the table, and as industries grapple with skills shortages, this demographic could be a vital resource.

Of course, there's also a flip side: will younger workers feel blocked by older employees remaining in the workforce longer? This might not be a pressing concern for certain sectors and industries, but for those that come with prestige and social standing, I can imagine individuals being reluctant to let go of their positions. This isn't really a hypothetical either; we already see it playing out "in miniature" in many settings, including academia. Professors, with the help of tenureship, are often insulated from the usual pressures that would lead to turnover in other industries. Combine this with high job satisfaction, and you're faced with people hanging on to the bitter end, stalling to vacate their position and stalling to make space for the next generation.

Regardless, policy changes will be critical in shaping how societies navigate these transitions. Tax reforms, universal access to lifelong learning, and incentives for flexible work arrangements are just a few of the measures that could help balance the needs of an aging population with economic sustainability.

We also have to consider questions around environmental sustainability. Are we really ready for a future where human lifespans stretch beyond 120 years? The idea of a world bursting at the seams with overpopulation is a common fear, for example, with visions of strained resources and an overburdened environment. But the reality might not be so straightforward.

On one hand, longer lifespans might exacerbate resource consumption. Older populations require more healthcare, energy, and infrastructure, and these demands could intensify environmental strain if sustainability isn't a core focus. Furthermore, as people live longer, global population numbers might temporarily spike, creating a period where more generations are alive simultaneously, increasing the consumption of finite resources like water, food, and energy.

But history provides a counterpoint. In many economically developed countries — such as Germany, Japan, and South Korea — longer lifespans have coincided with declining birth rates, leading to natural dips in population growth. The trend suggests that as societies grow wealthier and more advanced, they tend to stabilize or even shrink in population over time. Could this pattern hold globally? If so, longer lives might not necessarily mean overpopulation but rather a rebalancing of demographics, where fewer people live longer, healthier lives.

Whether longer lives lead to overpopulation or balance will depend, ultimately, on how we manage the transition. Can we adopt sustainable practices quickly enough? Will we prioritize equitable resource distribution?

Finally, we are left to confront the existential question: how long is too long? While the prospect of a life that spans centuries is alluring, could it not be the very brevity of life that gives it a sense of meaning and urgency? Knowing our time is finite spurs us to make intentional decisions, cherish fleeting moments, and push ourselves to achieve goals before our inevitable end.

Celebrated writer and poet, Jorge Luis Borges, made a case for this stance in one of his more famous works, *The Immortal*. Narrated by Marcus Flaminius Rufus, a Roman soldier, the story unfolds as a reflection on his extraordinary journey to discover the City of the Immortals. One night in Thebes, Rufus encounters a dying man who whispers of a river that grants eternal life. Drawn by the promise of immortality, Rufus embarks on an arduous trek into the heart of Africa.

The journey takes its toll. Desertion, betrayal, and the brutal desert landscape reduce his company to nothing. Alone and near death, Rufus stumbles upon a polluted stream and drinks deeply, unknowingly achieving his goal. Days later, he reaches the fabled City of the Immortals. What should be the pinnacle of his quest becomes a grotesque revelation. The city, with its dead-end staircases, inverted halls, and meaningless architecture, mirrors the chaos of immortality itself — it is a place devoid of purpose or reason, a monument to the futility of endless life.

Rufus learns that the city's builders, the Immortals, have destroyed their own original creation out of despair. Among them is Argos, a mute Troglodyte who, in time, reveals himself to be none other than Homer. Even the author of *The Iliad* has been reduced to silence, and Rufus is forced to recognize: the weight of eternal life renders all achievements hollow.

Borges' tale serves as a biting counterpoint to our ceaseless pursuit of life extension. Indeed, Rufus' journey reminds us that life's brevity is not purely a curse; it is also a gift. It is the limits of time that give our choices meaning and our accomplishments weight. Without these boundaries, the urgency to love, create, and strive fade into nothingness.

# References

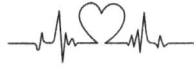

In this book, referencing is organized by chapter to facilitate a more streamlined and accessible reading experience. Each chapter includes its own set of references, allowing readers to easily locate sources relevant to the specific content discussed within that section. Readers are encouraged to consult the references at the end of each chapter for further exploration of the themes and concepts discussed.

## Prologue and Introduction

1.  Smith DG. The 7 Keys to Longevity. *The New York Times*. https://www.nytimes.com/2024/01/04/well/live/live-longer-health.html. Published January 4, 2024.

2.  Currey DR. An Ancient Bristlecone Pine Stand in Eastern Nevada. *Ecology*. 1965;46(4):564-566. doi:https://doi.org/10.2307/1934900

3.  Methuselah, a Bristlecone Pine is Thought to be the Oldest Living Organism on Earth. www.usda.gov. https://www.usda.gov/media/blog/2011/04/21/methuselah-bristlecone-pine-thought-be-oldest-living-organism-earth

4.  Matsumoto Y, Miglietta MP. Cellular reprogramming and immortality: Expression profiling reveals putative genes involved in Turritopsis dohrnii's life cycle reversal. Lavrov D, ed. *Genome Biology and Evolution*. 2021;13(7). doi:https://doi.org/10.1093/gbe/evab136

5. The Nobel Prize in Physiology or Medicine 2012. NobelPrize.org. Published 2012. https://www.nobelprize.org/prizes/medicine/2012/press-release/

## Chapter 1

6. Williams GC. PLEIOTROPY, NATURAL SELECTION, AND THE EVOLUTION OF SENESCENCE. Evolution. 1957;11(4):398-411. doi:https://doi.org/10.1111/j.1558-5646.1957.tb02911.x

7. Austad SN, Hoffman JM. Is antagonistic pleiotropy ubiquitous in aging biology? Evolution, Medicine, and Public Health. 2018;2018(1):287-294. doi:https://doi.org/10.1093/emph/eoy033

8. Mallapaty S. What is ageing? Even the field's researchers can't agree. Nature. 2024;636(8042):283-284. doi:https://doi.org/10.1038/d41586-024-03936-8

9. Gladyshev VN, Anderson B, Barlit H, et al. Disagreement on foundational principles of biological aging. Stover P, ed. PNAS Nexus. 2024;3(12). doi:https://doi.org/10.1093/pnasnexus/pgae499

10. Hou C. Grow fast, die young? Animals that invest in building high-quality biomaterials may slow aging and increase their lifespans. The Conversation. Published October 29, 2024.https://theconversation.com/grow-fast-die-young-animals-that-invest-in-building-high-quality-biomaterials-may-slow-aging-and-increase-their-lifespans-240517

11. Metcalfe NB, Monaghan P. Compensation for a bad start: grow now, pay later? *Trends in Ecology & Evolution.* 2001;16(5):254-260. doi:https://doi.org/10.1016/s0169-5347(01)02124-3

12. West GB, Brown JH, Enquist BJ. A general model for ontogenetic growth. *Nature.* 2001;413(6856):628-631. doi:https://doi.org/10.1038/35098076

13. Hou C. Energetic cost of biosynthesis is a missing link between growth and longevity in mammals. *Proceedings of the National Academy of Sciences.* 2024;121(20). doi:https://doi.org/10.1073/pnas.2315921121

14. Zhang Z, Schaefer C, Jiang W, et al. A panoramic view of cell population dynamics in mammalian aging. *Science (New York, NY).* Published online 2024:eadn3949. doi:https://doi.org/10.1126/science.adn3949

15. Shen X, Wang C, Zhou X, et al. Nonlinear dynamics of multi-omics profiles during human aging. *Nature Aging.* Published online August 14, 2024:1-16. doi:https://doi.org/10.1038/s43587-024-00692-2

## Chapter 2

16. López-Otín C, Blasco MA, Partridge L, Serrano M, Kroemer G. The Hallmarks of Aging. Cell. 2013;153(6):1194-1217. doi:https://doi.org/10.1016/j.cell.2013.05.039

17. López-Otín C, Blasco MA, Partridge L, Serrano M, Kroemer G. Hallmarks of aging: An expanding universe.

Cell. 2023;186(2):243-278.
doi:https://doi.org/10.1016/j.cell.2022.11.001

## Chapter 3

18. Schumacher B, Pothof J, Vijg J, Hoeijmakers JHJ. The central role of DNA damage in the ageing process. *Nature.* 2021;592(7856):695-703. doi:https://doi.org/10.1038/s41586-021-03307-7

19. Herr LM, Schaffer ED, Fuchs KF, Datta A, Brosh RM. Replication stress as a driver of cellular senescence and aging. *Communications Biology.* 2024;7(1):1-19. doi:https://doi.org/10.1038/s42003-024-06263-w

20. Vijg J. From DNA damage to mutations: All roads lead to aging. *Ageing Research Reviews.* 2021;68:101316. doi:https://doi.org/10.1016/j.arr.2021.101316

21. Haseltine WA. Why Do We Age? DNA Damage A Likely Cause. Forbes. Published February 13, 2024. Accessed November 12, 2024. https://www.forbes.com/sites/williamhaseltine/2024/02/13/why-do-we-age-dna-damage-a-likely-cause/

22. Haseltine WA. Molecular "Super Glue"? How Our Body Repairs Broken DNA. Forbes. https://www.forbes.com/sites/williamhaseltine/2024/02/25/molecular-super-glue-how-our-body-repairs-broken-dna/

23. Haseltine WA. Mitochondrial DNA And Aging: What's The Connection? *Forbes.* https://www.forbes.com/sites/williamhaseltine/2023/11/02/

mitochondrial-dna-and-aging-whats-the-connection/.
Published November 2, 2023.

24. Gyenis A, Chang J, Demmers JJPG, et al. Genome-wide RNA polymerase stalling shapes the transcriptome during aging. *Nature Genetics*. Published online January 19, 2023. doi:https://doi.org/10.1038/s41588-022-01279-6

25. Basky G. Newly discovered protein stops DNA damage. Phys.org. Published August 15, 2024. https://phys.org/news/2024-08-newly-protein-dna.html

26. Press C. Our cells are less likely to express longer genes as we age, researchers say. Medicalxpress.com. Published March 21, 2024. Accessed November 12, 2024. https://medicalxpress.com/news/2024-03-cells-longer-genes-age.html

27. McRae M. Mitochondria Dump DNA in The Brain, Potentially Cutting Years Off Our Lives. ScienceAlert. Published August 29, 2024. https://www.sciencealert.com/mitochondria-dump-dna-in-the-brain-potentially-cutting-years-off-our-lives

## Chapter 4

28. Gruber HJ, Semeraro MD, Renner W, Herrmann M. Telomeres and Age-Related Diseases. *Biomedicines*. 2021;9(10):1335. doi:https://doi.org/10.3390/biomedicines9101335

29. Stoneham K. Telomere Attrition: Hallmark of Aging #2. Oxford Healthspan® . Published January 13, 2023. Accessed November 12, 2024.

30. Shay JW, Wright WE. Hayflick, his limit, and cellular ageing. *Nature Reviews Molecular Cell Biology*. 2000;1(1):72-76. doi:Hayflick, his limit, and cellular ageing | Nature Reviews Molecular Cell Biology

31. Vaiserman A, Krasnienkov D. Telomere Length as a Marker of Biological Age: State-of-the-Art, Open Issues, and Future Perspectives. *Frontiers in Genetics*. 2021;11. doi:https://doi.org/10.3389/fgene.2020.630186

32. Schellnegger M, Lin AC, Hammer N, Kamolz LP. Physical Activity on Telomere Length as a Biomarker for Aging: A Systematic Review. *Sports Medicine - Open*. 2022;8(1). doi:https://doi.org/10.1186/s40798-022-00503-1

33. Haseltine WA. New Insights Into Aging: Not All Telomeres Are The Same. *Forbes*. https://www.forbes.com/sites/williamhaseltine/2024/08/08/new-insights-into-aging-not-all-telomeres-are-the-same/. Published August 8, 2024.

34. Haseltine WA. Telomeres, Or How Your DNA Shrinks Over Time. *Forbes*. https://www.forbes.com/sites/williamhaseltine/2024/07/16/telomeres-or-how-your-dna-shrinks-over-time/. Published July 16, 2024.

35. British Medical Journal. Shorter white blood cell telomeres linked to higher dementia risk. Medicalxpress.com. Published September 12, 2023. Accessed November 12, 2024. https://medicalxpress.com/news/2023-09-shorter-white-blood-cell-telomeres.html

36. Mannherz W, Agarwal S. Thymidine nucleotide metabolism controls human telomere length. *Nature Genetics.* 2023;55(4):568-580. doi:https://doi.org/10.1038/s41588-023-01339-5

37. Longevity Breakthrough: New Treatment Reverses Multiple Hallmarks of Aging. SciTechDaily. Published September 2, 2024. Accessed November 12, 2024. https://scitechdaily.com/longevity-breakthrough-new-treatment-reverses-multiple-hallmarks-of-aging/

## Chapter 5

38. Oxford Healthspan. Epigenetic Alterations: Hallmark of Aging #3. Oxford Healthspan® . Published January 14, 2023. Accessed November 12, 2024. https://oxfordhealthspan.com/blogs/aging-well/epigenetic-alterations-hallmark-of-aging-3

39. Why we Age: Epigenetic Alterations | Lifespan.io. www.lifespan.io. https://www.lifespan.io/topic/epigenetic-alterations/

40. Pouikli A, Tessarz P. Epigenetic alterations in stem cell ageing—a promising target for age-reversing interventions? *Briefings in Functional Genomics.* Published online March 19, 2021. doi:https://doi.org/10.1093/bfgp/elab010

41. Wang K, Liu H, Hu Q, et al. Epigenetic regulation of aging: implications for interventions of aging and diseases. *Signal Transduction and Targeted Therapy.* 2022;7(1):1-22. doi:https://doi.org/10.1038/s41392-022-01211-8

42. Dhar P, Moodithaya SS, Patil P. Epigenetic alterations—
The silent indicator for early aging and age-associated
health-risks. *AGING MEDICINE.* 2022;5(4).
doi:https://doi.org/10.1002/agm2.12236

43. Pereira B, Correia FP, Alves IA, et al. Epigenetic
reprogramming as a key to reverse ageing and increase
longevity. *Ageing Research Reviews.* 2024;95:102204.
doi:https://doi.org/10.1016/j.arr.2024.102204

44. National Institute on Aging. The epigenetics of aging:
What the body's hands of time tell us. *National Institutes of
Health.* https://www.nia.nih.gov/news/epigenetics-aging-
what-bodys-hands-time-tell-us. Published March 26, 2021.

45. Galkin F, Mamoshina P, Aliper A, de Magalhães JP,
Gladyshev VN, Zhavoronkov A. Biohorology and
biomarkers of aging: Current state-of-the-art, challenges
and opportunities. *Ageing Research Reviews.*
2020;60:101050.
doi:https://doi.org/10.1016/j.arr.2020.101050

46. Zhang Z, Christensen BC, Salas LA. Recalibrate concepts
of epigenetic aging clocks in human health. *Aging.*
Published online July 17, 2024.
doi:https://doi.org/10.18632/aging.206027

47. Haseltine WA. How Old Are You Really? New "Aging"
Clock Provides Clues. *Forbes.*
https://www.forbes.com/sites/williamhaseltine/2024/03/23/h
ow-old-are-you-really-new-aging-clock-provides-clues/.
Published March 23, 2024.

48. Could Epigenetic Age Acceleration, Not Actual Age, Better Predict How Well You Remember? - SBU News. SBU News - News & Features at Stony Brook University. Published October 30, 2023. Accessed November 12, 2024. https://news.stonybrook.edu/newsroom/press-release/medical/could-epigenetic-age-acceleration-not-actual-age-better-predict-how-well-you-remember/

49. Kabacik S, Lowe D, Fransen L, et al. The relationship between epigenetic age and the hallmarks of aging in human cells. *Nature Aging.* 2022;2(6):484-493. doi:https://doi.org/10.1038/s43587-022-00220-0

50. Health D. Time change for biological aging clocks: How immune cells shape our body's true age. Medicalxpress.com. Published January 8, 2024. Accessed November 12, 2024. https://medicalxpress.com/news/2024-01-biological-aging-clocks-immune-cells.html

51. Marra PS, Yamanashi T, Crutchley KJ, et al. Metformin use history and genome-wide DNA methylation profile: potential molecular mechanism for aging and longevity. *Aging.* 2023;15(3):601-616. doi:https://doi.org/10.18632/aging.204498

52. Brigham and Women's Hospital. New epigenetic clocks reinvent how we measure age. medicalxpress.com. https://medicalxpress.com/news/2024-02-epigenetic-clocks-reinvent-age.html

53. University of Pittsburgh. New study reveals molecular fingerprint of biological aging. Medicalxpress.com. Published March 8, 2024. Accessed November 12, 2024.

https://medicalxpress.com/news/2024-03-reveals-molecular-fingerprint-biological-aging.html

54. Qiu W, Chen H, Kaeberlein M, Lee SI. ExplaiNAble BioLogical Age (ENABL Age): an artificial intelligence framework for interpretable biological age. *The Lancet Healthy Longevity.* 2023;4(12):e711-e723. doi:https://doi.org/10.1016/s2666-7568(23)00189-7

55. Nusinovici S, Rim TH, Li H, et al. Application of a deep-learning marker for morbidity and mortality prediction derived from retinal photographs: a cohort development and validation study. *The Lancet Healthy Longevity.* 2024;5(10):100593. doi:https://doi.org/10.1016/S2666-7568(24)00089-8

56. Fang W, Chen S, Jin X, Liu S, Cao X, Liu B. Metabolomics in aging research: aging markers from organs. *Frontiers in cell and developmental biology.* 2023;11. doi:https://doi.org/10.3389/fcell.2023.1198794

57. M Austin Argentieri, Xiao S, Bennett D, et al. Proteomic aging clock predicts mortality and risk of common age-related diseases in diverse populations. *Nature Medicine.* Published online August 8, 2024. doi:https://doi.org/10.1038/s41591-024-03164-7

## Chapter 6

58. Fernandez S. Zen and the art of mitochondrial maintenance: The machinery of death makes a healthier life. Phys.org. Published November 8, 2023. Accessed

November 12, 2024. https://phys.org/news/2023-11-zen-art-mitochondrial-maintenance-machinery.html

59. Kulkarni AS, Gubbi S, Barzilai N. Benefits of Metformin in Attenuating the Hallmarks of Aging. *Cell Metabolism.* 2020;32(1):15-30. doi:https://doi.org/10.1016/j.cmet.2020.04.001

60. Amor C, Fernández-Maestre I, Chowdhury S, et al. Prophylactic and long-lasting efficacy of senolytic CAR T cells against age-related metabolic dysfunction. *Nature Aging.* Published online January 24, 2024:1-14. doi:https://doi.org/10.1038/s43587-023-00560-5

61. Hebrew University of Jerusalem. Researchers reveal secrets of aging beta cells and their ability to secrete insulin. Medicalxpress.com. Published June 4, 2024. Accessed November 12, 2024. https://medicalxpress.com/news/2024-06-reveal-secrets-aging-beta-cells.html

62. Llewellyn J, Hubbard SJ, Swift J. Translation is an emerging constraint on protein homeostasis in ageing. *Trends in Cell Biology.* 2024;34(8):646-656. doi:https://doi.org/10.1016/j.tcb.2024.02.001

63. Taylor RC, Dillin A. Aging as an Event of Proteostasis Collapse. *Cold Spring Harbor Perspectives in Biology.* 2011;3(5). doi:https://doi.org/10.1101/cshperspect.a004440

64. Hipp MS, Kasturi P, Hartl FU. The Proteostasis Network and Its Decline in Ageing. *Nature Reviews Molecular Cell Biology.* 2019;20(7):421-435. doi:https://doi.org/10.1038/s41580-019-0101-y

65. Why we Age: Loss of Proteostasis | Lifespan.io. www.lifespan.io. https://www.lifespan.io/topic/loss-of-proteostasis/

66. Klaips CL, Jayaraj GG, Hartl FU. Pathways of cellular proteostasis in aging and disease. *The Journal of Cell Biology.* 2018;217(1):51-63. doi:https://doi.org/10.1083/jcb.201709072

67. Thompson MA, De-Souza EA. A Year at the Forefront of Proteostasis and Aging. *Biology Open.* 2023;12(2). doi:https://doi.org/10.1242/bio.059750

68. Oxford Healthspan. Loss of Proteostasis: Hallmark of Aging #4. Oxford Healthspan® . Published January 16, 2023. Accessed November 12, 2024. https://oxfordhealthspan.com/blogs/aging-well/loss-of-proteostasis-hallmark-of-aging-4

## Chapter 7

69. Disabled Macroautophagy: Hallmark of Aging #10. Oxford Healthspan®. https://oxfordhealthspan.com/blogs/aging-well/disabled-macroautophagy-hallmark-of-aging-10

70. Nieto-Torres JL, Hansen M. Macroautophagy and aging: The impact of cellular recycling on health and longevity. *Molecular Aspects of Medicine.* 2021;82:101020. doi:https://doi.org/10.1016/j.mam.2021.101020

71. Wong ASL, Cheung ZH, Ip NY. Molecular machinery of macroautophagy and its deregulation in diseases. *Biochimica et Biophysica Acta (BBA) - Molecular Basis of*

*Disease.* 2011;1812(11):1490-1497.
doi:https://doi.org/10.1016/j.bbadis.2011.07.005

72. Johnson SC. Nutrient Sensing, Signaling and Ageing: The Role of IGF-1 and mTOR in Ageing and Age-Related Disease. *Sub-cellular biochemistry.* 2018;90:49-97. doi:https://doi.org/10.1007/978-981-13-2835-0_3

## Chapter 8

73. Stoneham K. Deregulated Nutrient Sensing: Hallmark of Aging #5. Oxford Healthspan® . Published March 21, 2024. Accessed November 12, 2024. https://oxfordhealthspan.com/blogs/aging-well/deregulated-nutrient-sensing-hallmark-of-aging-5

74. Yang K, Hou R, Zhao J, et al. Lifestyle effects on aging and CVD: A spotlight on the nutrient-sensing network. *Ageing Research Reviews.* 2023;92:102121. doi:https://doi.org/10.1016/j.arr.2023.102121

75. Why we Age: Deregulated Nutrient Sensing | Lifespan.io. www.lifespan.io. https://www.lifespan.io/topic/deregulated-nutrient-sensing/

76. Covarrubias AJ, Perrone R, Grozio A, Verdin E. NAD+ metabolism and its roles in cellular processes during ageing. *Nature Reviews Molecular Cell Biology.* 2020;22(2):119-141. doi:https://doi.org/10.1038/s41580-020-00313-x

77. Yao Y, Liu L, Guo G, Zeng Y, Ji JS. Interaction of Sirtuin 1 (SIRT1) candidate longevity gene and particulate matter (PM2.5) on all-cause mortality: a longitudinal cohort study

in China. *Environmental Health*. 2021;20(1). doi:https://doi.org/10.1186/s12940-021-00718-x

**Chapter 9**

78. Oxford Healthspan. Mitochondrial Dysfunction: Hallmark of Aging #6. Oxford Healthspan® . Published March 29, 2023. Accessed November 12, 2024. https://oxfordhealthspan.com/blogs/aging-well/mitochondrial-dysfunction-hallmark-of-aging-6

79. Srivastava S. The Mitochondrial Basis of Aging and Age-Related Disorders. *Genes*. 2017;8(12):398. doi:https://doi.org/10.3390/genes8120398

80. Amorim JA, Coppotelli G, Rolo AP, Palmeira CM, Ross JM, Sinclair DA. Mitochondrial and metabolic dysfunction in ageing and age-related diseases. *Nature Reviews Endocrinology*. 2022;18. doi:https://doi.org/10.1038/s41574-021-00626-7

81. Guo Y, Guan T, Shafiq K, et al. Mitochondrial dysfunction in aging. *Ageing Research Reviews*. 2023;88:101955-101955. doi:https://doi.org/10.1016/j.arr.2023.101955

82. Miwa S, Kashyap S, Chini E, von Zglinicki T. Mitochondrial dysfunction in cell senescence and aging. *Journal of Clinical Investigation*. 2022;132(13). doi:https://doi.org/10.1172/jci158447

83. Biology. Mdpi.com. Published 2024. Accessed November 12, 2024. https://www.mdpi.com/journal/biology/special_issues/Mitochondria

84. Why we Age: Mitochondrial Dysfunction | Lifespan.io. www.lifespan.io. https://www.lifespan.io/topic/mitochondrial-dysfunction/

## Chapter 10

85. Senescent immune cells spread damage throughout the aging body. National Institute on Aging. https://www.nia.nih.gov/news/senescent-immune-cells-spread-damage-throughout-aging-body

86. Herr LM, Schaffer ED, Fuchs KF, Datta A, Brosh RM. Replication stress as a driver of cellular senescence and aging. *Communications Biology*. 2024;7(1):1-19. doi:https://doi.org/10.1038/s42003-024-06263-w

87. von Kobbe C. Targeting senescent cells: approaches, opportunities, challenges. *Aging*. 2019;11(24). doi:https://doi.org/10.18632/aging.102557

88. Chaib S, Tchkonia T, Kirkland JL. Cellular senescence and senolytics: the path to the clinic. *Nature Medicine*. 2022;28(8):1556-1568. doi:https://doi.org/10.1038/s41591-022-01923-y

89. Haseltine WA. Old Cells Gone Bad: Fighting Senescent Cells With CAR-T Technology. *Forbes*. https://www.forbes.com/sites/williamhaseltine/2023/10/31/old-cells-gone-bad-fighting-senescent-cells-with-car-t-technology/?sh=35f086e2fbe8. Published October 31, 2023.

90. McHugh D, Sun B, Gutierrez-Muñoz C, et al. COPI vesicle formation and N-myristoylation are targetable

vulnerabilities of senescent cells. *Nature cell biology*. 2023;25(12):1804-1820. doi:https://doi.org/10.1038/s41556-023-01287-6

91. and S. Damage to cell membranes causes cell aging, finds new study. Phys.org. Published February 22, 2024. Accessed November 12, 2024. https://phys.org/news/2024-02-cell-membranes-aging.html

92. de P. How do we age? New probe can detect senescent cells in urine. Medicalxpress.com. Published February 28, 2024. Accessed November 12, 2024. https://medicalxpress.com/news/2024-02-age-probe-senescent-cells-urine.html

93. Center P. New study highlights senescent cell removal mechanisms of canagliflozin, a sodium glucose co-transporter 2 inhibitor. Medicalxpress.com. Published May 30, 2024. Accessed November 12, 2024. https://medicalxpress.com/news/2024-05-highlights-senescent-cell-mechanisms-canagliflozin.html

94. Herdy JR, Mertens J, Gage FH. Neuronal senescence may drive brain aging. *Science*. 2024;384(6703):1404-1406. doi:https://doi.org/10.1126/science.adi3450

95. UTSW study identifies RNA molecule that regulates cellular aging. Utsouthwestern.edu. Published July 17, 2024. Accessed November 12, 2024. https://www.utsouthwestern.edu/newsroom/articles/year-2024/july-rna-molecule-cellular-aging.html

96. Oxford Healthspan. Cellular Senescence: Hallmark of Aging #7. Oxford Healthspan® . Published April 24, 2023.

Accessed November 12, 2024.
https://oxfordhealthspan.com/blogs/aging-well/cellular-senescence-hallmark-of-aging-7

97. Why we Age: Cellular Senescence | Lifespan.io.
www.lifespan.io. https://www.lifespan.io/topic/cellular-senescence/

98. Senescent immune cells spread damage throughout the aging body. National Institute on Aging.
https://www.nia.nih.gov/news/senescent-immune-cells-spread-damage-throughout-aging-body

99. Shay JW, Wright WE. Hayflick, his limit, and cellular ageing. *Nature Reviews Molecular Cell Biology.*
2000;1(1):72-76. doi:https://doi.org/10.1038/35036093

100. Herr LM, Schaffer ED, Fuchs KF, Datta A, Brosh RM.
Replication stress as a driver of cellular senescence and aging. *Communications Biology.* 2024;7(1):1-19.
doi:https://doi.org/10.1038/s42003-024-06263-w

101. Di Micco R, Krizhanovsky V, Baker D, d'Adda di Fagagna F. Cellular Senescence in ageing: from Mechanisms to Therapeutic Opportunities. *Nature Reviews Molecular Cell Biology.* 2020;22(2):75-95.
doi:https://doi.org/10.1038/s41580-020-00314-w

102. McHugh D, Gil J. Senescence and aging: Causes, consequences, and Therapeutic Avenues. *The Journal of Cell Biology.* 2017;217(1):65-77.
doi:https://doi.org/10.1083/jcb.201708092

103. Zhang L, Pitcher LE, Yousefzadeh MJ, Niedernhofer LJ, Robbins PD, Zhu Y. Cellular senescence: a key therapeutic target in aging and diseases. *The Journal of Clinical Investigation*. 2022;132(15):e158450. doi:https://doi.org/10.1172/JCI158450

104. Witham MD, Antoneta Granic, Miwa S, Passos JF, Richardson GD, Sayer AA. New Horizons in cellular senescence for clinicians. *Age and Ageing*. 2023;52(7). doi:https://doi.org/10.1093/ageing/afad127

105. Reed R, Miwa S. Cellular Senescence and Ageing. *Subcellular biochemistry*. Published online January 1, 2023:139-173. doi:https://doi.org/10.1007/978-3-031-21410-3_7

106. Wissler Gerdes EO, Zhu Y, Weigand BM, et al. Chapter Eight - Cellular senescence in aging and age-related diseases: Implications for neurodegenerative diseases. ScienceDirect. Published January 1, 2020. https://www.sciencedirect.com/science/article/abs/pii/S0074774220300507

107. Pedro. Cellular senescence in normal physiology. *Science*. 2024;384(6702):1300-1301. doi:https://doi.org/10.1126/science.adj7050

108. Sun Y, Li Q, Kirkland JL. Targeting senescent cells for a healthier longevity: the roadmap for an era of global aging. 2022;1(2):103-119. doi:https://doi.org/10.1093/lifemedi/lnac030

109. Borghesan M, Hoogaars WMH, Varela-Eirin M, Talma N, Demaria M. A Senescence-Centric View of Aging:

Implications for Longevity and Disease. *Trends in Cell Biology*. 2020;30(10):777-791. doi:https://doi.org/10.1016/j.tcb.2020.07.002

110. Huang W, Hickson LJ, Eirin A, Kirkland JL, Lerman LO. Cellular senescence: the good, the bad and the unknown. *Nature Reviews Nephrology*. 2022;18. doi:https://doi.org/10.1038/s41581-022-00601-z

111. Kumar A, Thirumurugan K. Understanding cellular senescence: pathways involved, therapeutics and longevity aiding. *Cell Cycle*. 2023;22(20):2324-2345. doi:https://doi.org/10.1080/15384101.2023.2287929

## Chapter 11

112. Stem Cell Exhaustion: Hallmark of Aging #8. Oxford Healthspan®. https://oxfordhealthspan.com/blogs/aging-well/stem-cell-exhaustion-hallmark-of-aging-8

113. Rezazadeh S, Ellison-Hughes GM. Editorial: Stem cell exhaustion in aging. *Frontiers in Aging*. 2024;5. doi:https://doi.org/10.3389/fragi.2024.1433702

114. Lawton A, Tripodi N, Feehan J. Running on empty: Exploring stem cell exhaustion in geriatric musculoskeletal disease. *Maturitas*. 2024;188:108066. doi:https://doi.org/10.1016/j.maturitas.2024.108066

115. Stem Cell Exhaustion. www.lifespan.io. https://www.lifespan.io/topic/stem-cell-exhaustion/

116. Liu B, Qu J, Zhang W, Izpisua Belmonte JC, Liu GH. A stem cell aging framework, from mechanisms to

interventions. *Cell Reports*. 2022;41(3):111451.
doi:https://doi.org/10.1016/j.celrep.2022.111451

117. Wikipedia Contributors. Stem cell theory of aging.
Wikipedia. Published April 10, 2019.
https://en.wikipedia.org/wiki/Stem_cell_theory_of_aging

118. Lupatov A, Yarygin K, Telomeres T, Yegorov Y. Citation.
Published online 2022.
doi:https://doi.org/10.3390/biomedicines10102335

119. Hayflick Limit - an overview | ScienceDirect Topics.
www.sciencedirect.com.
https://www.sciencedirect.com/topics/biochemistry-
genetics-and-molecular-biology/hayflick-limit

120. Mi L, Hu J, Li N, et al. The Mechanism of Stem Cell
Aging. *Stem cell reviews and reports*. 2022;18(4):1281-
1293. doi:https://doi.org/10.1007/s12015-021-10317-5

## Chapter 12

121. Altered Intercellular Communication. www.lifespan.io.
https://www.lifespan.io/topic/altered-intercellular-
communication/

122. Oxford Healthspan. Altered Intracellular Communication:
Hallmark of Aging #9. Oxford Healthspan® . Published
June 27, 2023. Accessed November 12, 2024.
https://oxfordhealthspan.com/blogs/aging-well/altered-
intracellular-communication-hallmark-of-aging-9

123. Fafián-Labora JA, O'Loghlen A. Classical and
Nonclassical Intercellular Communication in Senescence

and Ageing. *Trends in Cell Biology*. 2020;30(8):628-639. doi:https://doi.org/10.1016/j.tcb.2020.05.003

## Chapter 13

124. Schumacher B, Pothof J, Vijg J, Hoeijmakers JHJ. The central role of DNA damage in the ageing process. *Nature*. 2021;592(7856):695-703. doi:https://doi.org/10.1038/s41586-021-03307-7

125. Herr LM, Schaffer ED, Fuchs KF, Datta A, Brosh RM. Replication stress as a driver of cellular senescence and aging. *Communications Biology*. 2024;7(1):1-19. doi:https://doi.org/10.1038/s42003-024-06263-w

126. Vijg J. From DNA damage to mutations: All roads lead to aging. *Ageing Research Reviews*. 2021;68:101316. doi:https://doi.org/10.1016/j.arr.2021.101316

127. Franceschi C, Garagnani P, Parini P, Giuliani C, Santoro A. Inflammaging: a new immune–metabolic viewpoint for age-related diseases. *Nature Reviews Endocrinology*. 2018;14(10):576-590. doi:https://doi.org/10.1038/s41574-018-0059-4

128. Liu Z, Liang Q, Ren Y, et al. Immunosenescence: molecular mechanisms and diseases. *Signal Transduction and Targeted Therapy*. 2023;8(1):1-16. doi:https://doi.org/10.1038/s41392-023-01451-2

129. Haseltine WA. Resolvins: Firefighters In The Battle Against Chronic Inflammation. *Forbes*. https://www.forbes.com/sites/williamhaseltine/2023/12/25/

resolvins-firefighters-in-the-battle-against-chronic-inflammation/. Published December 25, 2023.

130. Haseltine WA. Inflammation In The Brain Linked To Aging And Cognitive Decline. *Forbes*. https://www.forbes.com/sites/williamhaseltine/2023/11/13/inflammation-in-the-brain-linked-to-aging-and-cognitive-decline/. Published November 13, 2023.

131. Haseltine WA. What Causes Our Skin To Age? Inflammation A Likely Suspect. Forbes. Published October 4, 2023. Accessed November 12, 2024. https://www.forbes.com/sites/williamhaseltine/2023/10/04/what-causes-our-skin-to-age-inflammation-a-likely-suspect/

132. Haseltine WA. Forever Young? The Naked Mole Rat Teaches Scientists About Longevity. Forbes. https://www.forbes.com/sites/williamhaseltine/2023/10/17/forever-young-the-naked-mole-rat-teaches-scientists-about-longevity/

133. UK. Scientists discover switching off inflammatory protein leads to longer, healthier lifespans in mice. Medicalxpress.com. Published July 17, 2024. Accessed November 12, 2024. https://medicalxpress.com/news/2024-07-scientists-inflammatory-protein-longer-healthier.html

134. Rodrigues LP, Teixeira VR, Alencar-Silva T, et al. Hallmarks of aging and immunosenescence: Connecting the dots. *Cytokine & Growth Factor Reviews*. 2021;59:9-21. doi:https://doi.org/10.1016/j.cytogfr.2021.01.006

135. Haseltine WA. A Pomegranate A Day Keeps The Doctor Away? Researchers Rejuvenate Aging Immune Systems. *Forbes.* http://www.forbes.com/sites/williamhaseltine/2023/09/19/a-pomegranate-a-day-keeps-the-doctor-away-researchers-rejuvenate-aging-immune-systems/. Published September 19, 2023.

136. Haseltine WA. Can Your Immune System Be Rejuvenated? Yes, Says New Research. *Forbes.* https://www.forbes.com/sites/williamhaseltine/2024/04/19/can-your-immune-system-be-rejuvenated-yes-says-new-research/. Published April 19, 2024.

137. Immune resilience is key to a long and healthy life. National Institute on Aging. Published June 30, 2023. https://www.nia.nih.gov/news/immune-resilience-key-long-and-healthy-life

138. Society MP. Anti-aging drug rapamycin found to improve immune function through endolysosomes. Medicalxpress.com. Published February 28, 2024. Accessed November 12, 2024. https://medicalxpress.com/news/2024-02-anti-aging-drug-rapamycin-immune.html

139. Ledford H. How to make an old immune system young again. *Nature.* Published online March 27, 2024. doi:https://doi.org/10.1038/d41586-024-00871-6

140. Pilling G. Inflammation & "Inflammaging": Hallmark of Aging #11. Oxford Healthspan® . Published September 27, 2023. Accessed November 12, 2024.

https://oxfordhealthspan.com/blogs/aging-well/inflammation-inflammaging-hallmark-of-aging-11

141. Franceschi C, Garagnani P, Parini P, Giuliani C, Santoro A. Inflammaging: a new immune–metabolic viewpoint for age-related diseases. *Nature Reviews Endocrinology.* 2018;14(10):576-590. doi:https://doi.org/10.1038/s41574-018-0059-4

142. Baechle JJ, Chen N, Makhijani P, Winer S, Furman D, Winer DA. Chronic inflammation and the hallmarks of aging. *Molecular Metabolism.* 2023;74:101755. doi:https://doi.org/10.1016/j.molmet.2023.101755

143. Li X, Li C, Zhang W, Wang Y, Qian P, Huang H. Inflammation and aging: signaling pathways and intervention therapies. *Inflammation and aging: Signaling Pathways and Intervention Therapies.* 2023;8(1). doi:https://doi.org/10.1038/s41392-023-01502-8

144. Seegren PV, Harper LR, Downs TK, et al. Reduced mitochondrial calcium uptake in macrophages is a major driver of inflammaging. *Nature Aging.* 2023;3(7):796-812. doi:https://doi.org/10.1038/s43587-023-00436-8

145. Victorelli S, Salmonowicz H, Chapman J, et al. Apoptotic stress causes mtDNA release during senescence and drives the SASP. *Nature.* Published online October 11, 2023:1-10. doi:https://doi.org/10.1038/s41586-023-06621-4

## Chapter 14

146. Stoneham K. Gut Dysbiosis: Hallmark of Aging #12. Oxford Healthspan® . Published November 22, 2023.

Accessed November 12, 2024.
https://oxfordhealthspan.com/blogs/aging-well/gut-dysbiosis-hallmark-of-aging-12

147. Ragonnaud E, Biragyn A. Gut microbiota as the key controllers of "healthy" aging of elderly people. *Immunity & Ageing*. 2021;18(1). doi:https://doi.org/10.1186/s12979-020-00213-w

148. Dysbiosis - an overview | ScienceDirect Topics. Sciencedirect.com. Published 2017. https://www.sciencedirect.com/topics/medicine-and-dentistry/dysbiosis

149. Holmes A, Finger C, Morales-Scheihing D, Lee J, McCullough LD. Gut dysbiosis and age-related neurological diseases; an innovative approach for therapeutic interventions. *Translational Research*. 2020;226:39-56. doi:https://doi.org/10.1016/j.trsl.2020.07.012

150. Bosco N, Noti M. The aging gut microbiome and its impact on host immunity. *Genes & Immunity*. 2021;22. doi:https://doi.org/10.1038/s41435-021-00126-8

151. Ghosh TS, Shanahan F, O'Toole PW. The gut microbiome as a modulator of healthy ageing. *Nature Reviews Gastroenterology & Hepatology*. 2022;19. doi:https://doi.org/10.1038/s41575-022-00605-x

152. Haran JP, McCormick BA. Aging, Frailty, and the Microbiome—How Dysbiosis Influences Human Aging and Disease. *Gastroenterology*. 2021;160(2):507-523. doi:https://doi.org/10.1053/j.gastro.2020.09.060

153. Molinero N, Antón-Fernández A, Hernández F, Ávila J, Bartolomé B, Moreno-Arribas MV. Gut Microbiota, an Additional Hallmark of Human Aging and Neurodegeneration. *Neuroscience*. Published online March 2023. doi:https://doi.org/10.1016/j.neuroscience.2023.02.014

154. Haseltine WA. Can We Turn Back The Clock? Parabiosis Research Suggests Yes. *Forbes*. https://www.forbes.com/sites/williamhaseltine/2023/09/01/can-we-turn-back-the-clock-parabiosis-research-suggests-yes/. Published September 1, 2023.

## Chapter 15

155. Zhang Y, Murata S, Schmidt-Mende K, Ebeling M, Modig K. Do people reach 100 by surviving, delaying, or avoiding diseases? A life course comparison of centenarians and non-centenarians from the same birth cohorts. *GeroScience*. Published online August 30, 2024. doi:https://doi.org/10.1007/s11357-024-01330-w

156. Reed P. Prevention Is Still the Best Medicine - News & Events | odphp.health.gov. Health.gov. Published 2024. https://odphp.health.gov/news/202401/prevention-still-best-medicine

157. Levine S, Malone E, Lekiachvili A, Briss P. Health care industry insights: Why the use of preventive services is still low. *Preventing Chronic Disease*. 2019;16(16). doi:https://doi.org/10.5888/pcd16.180625

158.The Conversation. Diet-related diseases: U.S. medical training is failing to address nation's #1 killer. Study Finds. Published September 30, 2024. Accessed December 3, 2024. https://studyfinds.org/diet-diseases-medical-training/

159.Mokdad AH, Ballestros K, Echko M, et al. The State of US Health, 1990-2016. *JAMA.* 2018;319(14):1444. doi:https://doi.org/10.1001/jama.2018.0158

160.Adams KM, Kohlmeier M, Zeisel SH. Nutrition education in U.S. medical schools: latest update of a national survey. *Academic medicine : journal of the Association of American Medical Colleges.* 2010;85(9):1537-1542. doi:https://doi.org/10.1097/ACM.0b013e3181eab71b

161.Zhang Y, Murata S, Schmidt-Mende K, Ebeling M, Modig K. Do people reach 100 by surviving, delaying, or avoiding diseases? A life course comparison of centenarians and non-centenarians from the same birth cohorts. *GeroScience.* Published online August 30, 2024. doi:https://doi.org/10.1007/s11357-024-01330-w

162.Engberg H, Oksuzyan A, Jeune B, Vaupel JW, Christensen K. Centenarians - a useful model for healthy aging? A 29-year follow-up of hospitalizations among 40 000 Danes born in 1905. *Aging Cell.* 2009;8(3):270-276. doi:https://doi.org/10.1111/j.1474-9726.2009.00474.x

163.Willcox DC, Willcox BJ, Wang NC, He Q, Rosenbaum M, Suzuki M. Life at the Extreme Limit: Phenotypic Characteristics of Supercentenarians in Okinawa. *The Journals of Gerontology: Series A.* 2008;63(11):1201-1208. doi:https://doi.org/10.1093/gerona/63.11.1201

164. Clerencia-Sierra M, Ioakeim-Skoufa I, Poblador-Plou B, et al. Do Centenarians Die Healthier than Younger Elders? A Comparative Epidemiological Study in Spain. *Journal of Clinical Medicine.* 2020;9(5):1563. doi:https://doi.org/10.3390/jcm9051563

## Chapter 16

165. Katz B. 2,000-Year-Old Texts Reveal the First Emperor of China's Quest for Eternal Life. Smithsonian Magazine. Published December 29, 2017. https://www.smithsonianmag.com/smart-news/2000-year-old-texts-reveal-first-emperor-chinas-quest-eternal-life-180967671/

166. Burman E. The Art of Not Dying | Edward Burman. Lapham's Quarterly. Published August 8, 2018. https://www.laphamsquarterly.org/roundtable/art-not-dying

167. Zhao G, Zhang W, Duan Z, et al. Mercury as a Geophysical Tracer Gas - Emissions from the Emperor Qin Tomb in Xi'an Studied by Laser Radar. *Scientific Reports.* 2020;10(1):10414. doi:https://doi.org/10.1038/s41598-020-67305-x

168. Konstantine Panegyres. The secret to living a longer, healthier life — according to the ancients. Medicalxpress.com. Published November 6, 2024. Accessed December 3, 2024. https://medicalxpress.com/news/2024-11-secret-longer-healthier-life-ancients.html

169. Henderson J. *Letters, Volume I: Books 1-7.*
https://www.loebclassics.com/view/LCL055/1969/volume.
xml

170. Hygiene, Volume II. Loeb Classical Library. Published
2018. Accessed December 3, 2024.
https://www.loebclassics.com/view/LCL536/2018/volume.
xml

171. Method of Medicine, Volume III. Loeb Classical Library.
Published 2024. Accessed December 3, 2024.
https://www.loebclassics.com/view/LCL518/2011/volume.
xml

## Chapter 17

172. Senay Boztas. Europe's champion sitters: even the sporty
Dutch are falling victim to "chair-use disorder." the
Guardian. Published March 17, 2024.
https://www.theguardian.com/lifeandstyle/2024/mar/17/eu
ropes-champion-sitters-even-the-sporty-dutch-are-falling-
victim-to-chair-use-disorder

173. Haseltine WA. How Exercise Helps Fight Alzheimer's
Disease. *Forbes.*
https://www.forbes.com/sites/williamhaseltine/2023/09/21/
how-exercise-helps-fight-alzheimers-disease/. Published
September 21, 2023.

174. Garcia L, Pearce M, Abbas A, et al. Non-occupational
physical activity and risk of cardiovascular disease, cancer
and mortality outcomes: a dose–response meta-analysis of
large prospective studies. *British Journal of Sports*

*Medicine.* 2023;57(15).
doi:https://doi.org/10.1136/bjsports-2022-105669

175. Oup.com. Published 2024.
https://academic.oup.com/biomedgerontology/advance-article-abstract/doi/10.1093/gerona/glad257/7390642

176. Wiley. Chronic inflammation and inactivity may affect age-related changes in gene and protein expression in skeletal muscle. Medicalxpress.com. Published February 21, 2024. https://medicalxpress.com/news/2024-02-chronic-inflammation-inactivity-affect-age.html

177. London KC. Muscle health may be informed by activity level rather than aging process. Medicalxpress.com. Published March 21, 2024. https://medicalxpress.com/news/2024-03-muscle-health-aging.html

178. Boone M. Regular exercise prevents DNA damage with aging. Medicalxpress.com. Published April 8, 2024. https://medicalxpress.com/news/2024-04-regular-dna-aging.html

179. Public. Study in women shows significant link between regular exercise during middle-age and physical health in later life. Medicalxpress.com. Published May 2, 2024. https://medicalxpress.com/news/2024-05-women-significant-link-regular-middle.html

180. Touchstone LA. Nerves prompt muscle to release factors that boost brain health, study finds. Medicalxpress.com. Published May 6, 2024.

https://medicalxpress.com/news/2024-05-nerves-prompt-muscle-factors-boost.html

181. First Steps Toward a Whole-Body Map of Molecular Responses to Exercise. PNNL. Published May 2024. https://www.pnnl.gov/news-media/first-steps-toward-whole-body-map-molecular-responses-exercise

182. Dolan EW. High-intensity interval training boosts cognitive function, with effects lasting up to five years. PsyPost - Psychology News. Published August 25, 2024. https://www.psypost.org/high-intensity-interval-training-boosts-cognitive-function-with-effects-lasting-up-to-five-years/

183. Nilsson MI, Tarnopolsky MA. Mitochondria and Aging— The Role of Exercise as a Countermeasure. *Biology*. 2019;8(2):40. doi:https://doi.org/10.3390/biology8020040

184. Veerman L, Tarp J, Wijaya R, et al. Physical activity and life expectancy: a life-table analysis. *British Journal of Sports Medicine*. Published online November 14, 2024:bjsports-2024-108125. doi:https://doi.org/10.1136/bjsports-2024-108125

185. Li Y, Wang K, Guliyeerke Jigeer, et al. Healthy Lifestyle and the Likelihood of Becoming a Centenarian. *JAMA Network Open*. 2024;7(6):e2417931-e2417931. doi:https://doi.org/10.1001/jamanetworkopen.2024.17931

## Chapter 18

186. Haseltine WA. You Are What You Eat? How Diet Boosts Brain Health. *Forbes*.

https://www.forbes.com/sites/williamhaseltine/2024/03/02/
you-are-what-you-eat-how-diet-boosts-brain-health/.
Published March 2, 2024.

187. Brandhorst S, Levine ME, Wei M, et al. Fasting-
     mimicking diet causes hepatic and blood markers changes
     indicating reduced biological age and disease risk. *Nature
     Communications.* 2024;15(1):1309.
     doi:https://doi.org/10.1038/s41467-024-45260-9

188. Columbia. Calorie restriction slows pace of aging in
     healthy adults. Medicalxpress.com. Published February 9,
     2023. Accessed November 12, 2024.
     https://medicalxpress.com/news/2023-02-calorie-
     restriction-pace-aging-healthy.html

189. Madhavan SS, Roa Diaz S, Peralta S, et al. β-
     hydroxybutyrate is a metabolic regulator of proteostasis in
     the aged and Alzheimer disease brain. *Cell Chemical
     Biology.* Published online December 2024.
     doi:https://doi.org/10.1016/j.chembiol.2024.11.001

190. Fadnes LT, Celis-Morales C, Økland JM, et al. Life
     expectancy can increase by up to 10 years following
     sustained shifts towards healthier diets in the United
     Kingdom. *Nature Food.* 2023;4(11):961-965.
     doi:https://doi.org/10.1038/s43016-023-00868-w

191. Zhu K, Li R, Yao P, et al. Proteomic signatures of healthy
     dietary patterns are associated with lower risks of major
     chronic diseases and mortality. *Nature Food.* Published
     online September 27, 2024.
     doi:https://doi.org/10.1038/s43016-024-01059-x

192. Eating less can lead to a longer life: massive study in mice shows why. *Naturecom*. Published online October 9, 2024. doi:https://doi.org/10.1038/d41586-024-03277-6

193. Kozlov M. The surprising cause of fasting's regenerative powers. *Nature*. Published online August 21, 2024. doi:https://doi.org/10.1038/d41586-024-02700-2

194. on S. Signs of accelerated aging found in brains of individuals with alcohol use disorder. Medicalxpress.com. Published January 26, 2024. Accessed November 12, 2024. https://medicalxpress.com/news/2024-01-aging-brains-individuals-alcohol-disorder.html

195. Salvestrini V, Sell C, Lorenzini A. Obesity May Accelerate the Aging Process. *Frontiers in Endocrinology*. 2019;10. doi:https://doi.org/10.3389/fendo.2019.00266

196. Coast S. Avoid inflammatory food to help save aging muscles, says researcher. Medicalxpress.com. Published January 22, 2024. Accessed November 12, 2024. https://medicalxpress.com/news/2024-01-inflammatory-food-aging-muscles.html

197. Journal BM. Consistent evidence links ultra-processed food to over 30 damaging health outcomes. medicalxpress.com. https://medicalxpress.com/news/2024-02-evidence-links-ultra-food-health.html

198. Luo Y, Stent S. Smoking's lasting effect on the immune system. *Nature*. Published online February 14, 2024. doi:https://doi.org/10.1038/d41586-024-00232-3

199. Institute for Health Metrics and Evaluation. GBD Compare. VizHub. Published 2021. https://vizhub.healthdata.org/gbd-compare/

200. Brandhorst S, Levine ME, Wei M, et al. Fasting-mimicking diet causes hepatic and blood markers changes indicating reduced biological age and disease risk. *Nature Communications.* 2024;15(1):1309. doi:https://doi.org/10.1038/s41467-024-45260-9

201. Columbia. Calorie restriction slows pace of aging in healthy adults. Medicalxpress.com. Published February 9, 2023. https://medicalxpress.com/news/2023-02-calorie-restriction-pace-aging-healthy.html

202. Zhu K, Li R, Yao P, et al. Proteomic signatures of healthy dietary patterns are associated with lower risks of major chronic diseases and mortality. *Nature Food.* Published online September 27, 2024. doi:https://doi.org/10.1038/s43016-024-01059-x

203. Eating less can lead to a longer life: massive study in mice shows why. *Naturecom.* Published online October 9, 2024. doi:https://doi.org/10.1038/d41586-024-03277-6

204. Kozlov M. The surprising cause of fasting's regenerative powers. *Nature.* Published online August 21, 2024. doi:https://doi.org/10.1038/d41586-024-02700-2

205. Uribarri J, Woodruff S, Goodman S, et al. Advanced Glycation End Products in Foods and a Practical Guide to Their Reduction in the Diet. *Journal of the American Dietetic Association.* 2010;110(6):911-916.e12. doi:https://doi.org/10.1016/j.jada.2010.03.018

206. Fadnes LT, Celis-Morales C, Økland JM, et al. Life expectancy can increase by up to 10 years following sustained shifts towards healthier diets in the United Kingdom. *Nature Food.* 2023;4(11):961-965. doi:https://doi.org/10.1038/s43016-023-00868-w

207. NHS. The Eatwell Guide. NHS. Published 2022. https://www.nhs.uk/live-well/eat-well/food-guidelines-and-food-labels/the-eatwell-guide/

208. Kenny L. Spermidine, a Calorie Restriction Mimetic for Longevity. Oxford Healthspan® . Published August 26, 2022. Accessed December 3, 2024. https://oxfordhealthspan.com/blogs/aging-well/spermidine-a-calorie-restriction-mimetic-for-longevity

## Chapter 19

209. Ludwig. Study shows good sleep stimulates the immune system. Medicalxpress.com. Published March 8, 2024. Accessed November 12, 2024. https://medicalxpress.com/news/2024-03-good-immune.html

210. Haseltine WA. Sleep Promotes Brain Health. Now We Know Why. *Forbes.* https://www.forbes.com/sites/williamhaseltine/2024/03/08/sleep-promotes-brain-health-now-we-know-why/. Published March 8, 2024.

211. University of Oulu. Research shows irregular sleep rhythm challenges the health of middle-aged people. Medicalxpress.com. Published January 24, 2024.

https://medicalxpress.com/news/2024-01-irregular-rhythm-health-middle-aged.html

212.Balter LJT, Axelsson J. Sleep and subjective age: protect your sleep if you want to feel young. *PubMed.* 2024;291(2019):20240171-20240171. doi:https://doi.org/10.1098/rspb.2024.0171

213.Sabia S, Fayosse A, Dumurgier J, et al. Association of sleep duration in middle and old age with incidence of dementia. *Nature Communications.* 2021;12(1):2289. doi:https://doi.org/10.1038/s41467-021-22354-2

214.Rihm JS, Menz MM, Schultz H, et al. Sleep Deprivation Selectively Upregulates an Amygdala–Hypothalamic Circuit Involved in Food Reward. *The Journal of Neuroscience.* 2018;39(5):888-899. doi:https://doi.org/10.1523/jneurosci.0250-18.2018

215.Oup.com. Published 2024. Accessed December 3, 2024. https://academic.oup.com/qjmed/article-abstract/117/3/177/7311739

216.Oup.com. Published 2024. Accessed December 3, 2024. https://academic.oup.com/sleep/article/47/1/zsad253/7280269

217.Napoli N. Getting Good Sleep Could Add Years to Your Life. American College of Cardiology. Published February 23, 2023. https://www.acc.org/About-ACC/Press-Releases/2023/02/22/21/35/Getting-Good-Sleep-Could-Add-Years-to-Your-Life

218. Jean-Louis G, Grandner MA, Pandi-Perumal SR. Sleep Health and Longevity—Considerations for Personalizing Existing Recommendations. *JAMA Network Open.* 2021;4(9):e2124387. doi:https://doi.org/10.1001/jamanetworkopen.2021.24387

## Chapter 20

219. Johnson A, Gomez C. Stress is weathering our bodies from the inside out. Washington Post. Published October 17, 2023. https://www.washingtonpost.com/health/interactive/2023/stress-chronic-illness-aging/

220. Wu Z, Qu J, Zhang W, Liu G. Stress, epigenetics, and aging: Unraveling the intricate crosstalk. *Molecular Cell.* Published online November 1, 2023. doi:https://doi.org/10.1016/j.molcel.2023.10.006

221. Poganik JR, Zhang B, Baht GS, et al. Biological age is increased by stress and restored upon recovery. *Cell Metabolism.* 2023;35(5):S1550-4131(23)000931. doi:https://doi.org/10.1016/j.cmet.2023.03.015

222. Harvanek ZM, Fogelman N, Xu K, Sinha R. Psychological and biological resilience modulates the effects of stress on epigenetic aging. *Translational Psychiatry.* 2021;11(1):1-9. doi:https://doi.org/10.1038/s41398-021-01735-7

223. Oup.com. Published 2024. Accessed December 3, 2024. https://academic.oup.com/biomedgerontology/article-abstract/69/Suppl_1/S10/586943

224. Lu S. https://www.apa.org/monitor/2014/10/chronic-stress. www.apa.org. Published October 2014. https://www.apa.org/monitor/2014/10/chronic-stress

225. McManus E, Haroon H, Duncan NW, Elliott R, Muhlert N. The effects of stress across the lifespan on the brain, cognition and mental health: A UK biobank study. *Neurobiology of Stress*. 2022;18:100447. doi:https://doi.org/10.1016/j.ynstr.2022.100447

226. Toda T, Parylak SL, Linker SB, Gage FH. The role of adult hippocampal neurogenesis in brain health and disease. *Molecular Psychiatry*. 2018;24(1):67-87. doi:https://doi.org/10.1038/s41380-018-0036-2

227. Harvard Health Publishing. A 20-minute nature break relieves stress. Harvard Health. Published July 1, 2019. https://www.health.harvard.edu/mind-and-mood/a-20-minute-nature-break-relieves-stress

## Chapter 21

228. Haseltine WA. A Quick Guide To "Social Health," And Why You Should Care About It. *Forbes*. https://www.forbes.com/sites/williamhaseltine/2024/06/18/a-quick-guide-to-social-health-and-why-you-should-care-about-it/. Published June 18, 2024.

229. Haseltine WA. Battling Loneliness: The New Public Health Crisis. Forbes. Published May 29, 2024. https://www.forbes.com/sites/williamhaseltine/2024/05/29/battling-loneliness-the-new-public-health-crisis/

230. GOV.UK. Government's work on tackling loneliness. GOV.UK. Published 2022. https://www.gov.uk/guidance/governments-work-on-tackling-loneliness

231. Preparatory Meeting of the Collaborative Platform for Loneliness and Isolation Measures (Provisional Name) (The Prime Minister in Action) | Prime Minister of Japan and His Cabinet. japan.kantei.go.jp. https://japan.kantei.go.jp/99_suga/actions/202109/_00033.html

232. Office of the Assistant Secretary for Health (OASH). New Surgeon General Advisory Raises Alarm about the Devastating Impact of the Epidemic of Loneliness and Isolation in the United States. U.S. Department of Health and Human Services. Published May 3, 2023. https://www.hhs.gov/about/news/2023/05/03/new-surgeon-general-advisory-raises-alarm-about-devastating-impact-epidemic-loneliness-isolation-united-states.html

233. World Health Organization. WHO launches commission to foster social connection. www.who.int. Published November 15, 2023. https://www.who.int/news/item/15-11-2023-who-launches-commission-to-foster-social-connection

234. Graham EK, Beck ED, Jackson K, et al. Do We Become More Lonely With Age? A Coordinated Data Analysis of Nine Longitudinal Studies. *Psychological science*. 2024;35(6). doi:https://doi.org/10.1177/09567976241242037

235. Moeyersons M, De Vliegher K, Huyghe B, De Groof S, Milisen K, de Casterlé BD. "Living in a shrinking world"—The experience of loneliness among community-dwelling older people with reduced mobility: a qualitative grounded theory approach. *BMC Geriatrics.* 2022;22(1). doi:https://doi.org/10.1186/s12877-022-02998-5

236. Huang AR, Thomas, Rebok GW, Swenor BK, Deal JA. Hearing and vision impairment and social isolation over 8 years in community-dwelling older adults. *BMC public health (Online).* 2024;24(1). doi:https://doi.org/10.1186/s12889-024-17730-8

237. Reed N, Morales E, Myers C, et al. Prevalence of Hearing Loss and Hearing Aid Use Among US Medicare Beneficiaries Aged 71 Years and Older. *JAMA network open.* 2023;6(7):e2326320-e2326320. doi:https://doi.org/10.1001/jamanetworkopen.2023.26320

238. Infurna FJ, Dey Y, Tita Gonzalez Avilés, Grimm KJ, Lachman ME, Gerstorf D. Loneliness in midlife: Historical increases and elevated levels in the United States compared with Europe. *American psychologist/The American psychologist.* Published online March 18, 2024. doi:https://doi.org/10.1037/amp0001322

239. Infurna FJ. Loneliness can kill, and new research shows middle-aged Americans are particularly vulnerable. The Conversation. Published April 5, 2024. https://theconversation.com/loneliness-can-kill-and-new-research-shows-middle-aged-americans-are-particularly-vulnerable-225321

240. Algren MH, Ekholm O, Nielsen L, Ersbøll AK, Bak CK, Andersen PT. Social isolation, loneliness, socioeconomic status, and health-risk behaviour in deprived neighbourhoods in Denmark: A cross-sectional study. *SSM - Population Health*. 2020;10(10):100546. doi:https://doi.org/10.1016/j.ssmph.2020.100546

241. Confronting Poverty. America's Poor Are Worse Off Than Elsewhere. Confronting Poverty. Published 2024. https://confrontingpoverty.org/poverty-facts-and-myths/americas-poor-are-worse-off-than-elsewhere/

242. *Government at a Glance 2021 Country Fact Sheet.* https://www.oecd.org/gov/gov-at-a-glance-2021-united-states.pdf

243. Galindo Y. Walkable Neighborhoods Help Adults Socialize, Increase Community. today.ucsd.edu. Published June 20, 2023. https://today.ucsd.edu/story/walkable-neighborhoods-help-adults-socialize-increase-community

244. National Academies of Sciences. *Social Isolation and Loneliness in Older Adults: Opportunities for the Health Care System.* National Academies Press; 2020. https://nap.nationalacademies.org/catalog/25663/social-isolation-and-loneliness-in-older-adults-opportunities-for-the

245. Manemann SM, Chamberlain AM, Roger VL, et al. Perceived Social Isolation and Outcomes in Patients With Heart Failure. *Journal of the American Heart Association*. 2018;7(11). doi:https://doi.org/10.1161/jaha.117.008069

246. David Matthew Doyle, Link BG. On social health: history, conceptualization, and population patterning. *Health Psychology Review.* Published online February 13, 2024:1-30. doi:https://doi.org/10.1080/17437199.2024.2314506

247. BridgetGWS. Governments Ramp Up the War on Loneliness. Global Wellness Summit. Published May 9, 2023. https://www.globalwellnesssummit.com/blog/governments-ramp-up-the-war-on-loneliness/

248. Morrish N, Choudhury S, Medina-Lara A. What works in interventions targeting loneliness: a systematic review of intervention characteristics. *BMC public health.* 2023;23(1):2214. doi:https://doi.org/10.1186/s12889-023-17097-2

249. Hoang P, King JA, Moore S, et al. Interventions Associated With Reduced Loneliness and Social Isolation in Older Adults. *JAMA Network Open.* 2022;5(10). doi:https://doi.org/10.1001/jamanetworkopen.2022.36676

250. Matsuda N, Murata S, Torizawa K, et al. Association Between Public Transportation Use and Loneliness Among Urban Elderly People Who Stop Driving. *Gerontology and Geriatric Medicine.* 2019;5:233372141985129. doi:https://doi.org/10.1177/2333721419851293

251. Astell-Burt T, Hartig T, Putra IGNE, Walsan R, Dendup T, Feng X. Green space and loneliness: A systematic review with theoretical and methodological guidance for future research. *Science of The Total Environment.*

2022;847:157521.
doi:https://doi.org/10.1016/j.scitotenv.2022.157521

252. Tomova L, Wang KL, Thompson T, et al. Acute social isolation evokes midbrain craving responses similar to hunger. *Nature Neuroscience.* 2020;23(12):1597-1605. doi:https://doi.org/10.1038/s41593-020-00742-z

253. Zhang S. The Plan to Stop Every Respiratory Virus at Once. The Atlantic. Published September 7, 2021. https://www.theatlantic.com/health/archive/2021/09/coronavirus-pandemic-ventilation-rethinking-air/620000/

## Chapter 22

254. U.S. Department of Health and Human Services. Social determinants of health and older adults. health.gov. Published May 13, 2024. https://health.gov/our-work/national-health-initiatives/healthy-aging/social-determinants-health-and-older-adults

255. Columbia. More schooling is linked to slowed aging and increased longevity. Medicalxpress.com. Published March 2024. Accessed November 12, 2024. https://medicalxpress.com/news/2024-03-schooling-linked-aging-longevity.html

256. Achenbach J. Life expectancy in U.S. is falling amid surges in chronic illness. Washington Post. Published October 3, 2023. Accessed November 12, 2024. https://www.washingtonpost.com/health/interactive/2023/american-life-expectancy-dropping/?itid=hp-top-table-main_p001_f001&itid=lk_interstitial_manual_34

257. Shipman M. Greener neighborhoods can protect us — at the cellular level. Phys.org. Published October 18, 2023. Accessed November 12, 2024. https://phys.org/news/2023-10-greener-neighborhoods-usat-cellular.html

258. Lawler D, Cortes I. Heat, disease, air pollution: How climate change impacts health. phys.org. https://phys.org/news/2023-11-disease-air-pollution-climate-impacts.html

259. London. First comprehensive global analysis shows action on emissions can bring huge health benefits. Phys.org. Published November 21, 2023. Accessed November 12, 2024. https://phys.org/news/2023-11-comprehensive-global-analysis-action-emissions.html

260. National Cancer Institute. PFAS Exposure and Risk of Cancer - National Cancer Institute. dceg.cancer.gov. Published October 15, 2020. https://dceg.cancer.gov/research/what-we-study/pfas

261. Singh GK, Lee H. Marked Disparities in Life Expectancy by Education, Poverty Level, Occupation, and Housing Tenure in the United States, 1997-2014. *International Journal of Maternal and Child Health and AIDS*. 2021;10(1):7-18. doi:https://doi.org/10.21106/ijma.402

262. Dutta-Gupta I. The Enduring Effects of Childhood Poverty. CLASP. Published August 14, 2023. https://www.clasp.org/blog/the-enduring-effects-of-childhood-poverty/

263. Dwyer-Lindgren L, Baumann MM, Li Z, et al. Ten Americas: a systematic analysis of life expectancy

disparities in the USA. *The Lancet.* Published online November 2024. doi:https://doi.org/10.1016/s0140-6736(24)01495-8

264. Office of Disease Prevention and Health Promotion. Poverty - Healthy People 2030. Health.gov. Published 2021. https://odphp.health.gov/healthypeople/priority-areas/social-determinants-health/literature-summaries/poverty

265. Aller MA, Arias N, Peral I, García-Higarza S, Arias JL, Arias J. Embrionary way to create a fatty liver in portal hypertension. *World Journal of Gastrointestinal Pathophysiology.* 2017;8(2):39. doi:https://doi.org/10.4291/wjgp.v8.i2.39

266. Schanzenbach D, Nunn R, Bauer L. *The Hamilton Project • Brookings Advancing Opportunity, Prosperity, and Growth the Changing Landscape of American Life Expectancy.*; 2016. https://www.hamiltonproject.org/assets/files/changing_landscape_american_life_expectancy.pdf

267. State of the Region's Health 2023 Update. RPA. https://rpa.org/work/reports/state-of-the-regions-health-2023-update

268. Gloria, Aiello AE, Caspi A, et al. Educational Mobility, Pace of Aging, and Lifespan Among Participants in the Framingham Heart Study. *JAMA Network Open.* 2024;7(3):e240655-e240655. doi:https://doi.org/10.1001/jamanetworkopen.2024.0655

269. Balaj M, Henson C, Aronsson A, et al. Effects of education on adult mortality: a global systematic review and meta-analysis. *The Lancet Public Health*. 2024;9(3). doi:https://doi.org/10.1016/s2468-2667(23)00306-7

270. The Lancet Public Health. Education: a neglected social determinant of health. *The Lancet Public Health*. 2020;5(7):361. doi:https://doi.org/10.1016/s2468-2667(20)30144-4

271. Tawakol A, Osborne MT, Wang Y, et al. Stress-Associated Neurobiological Pathway Linking Socioeconomic Disparities to Cardiovascular Disease. *Journal of the American College of Cardiology*. 2019;73(25):3243-3255. doi:https://doi.org/10.1016/j.jacc.2019.04.042

272. Cohen AK, Nussbaum J, Weintraub MLR, Nichols CR, Yen IH. Association of Adult Depression With Educational Attainment, Aspirations, and Expectations. *Preventing Chronic Disease*. 2020;17. doi:https://doi.org/10.5888/pcd17.200098

273. Prochaska M. Children's Legal Rights Journal Statistically Speaking: Evaluation of the Becoming a Man (B.A.M.) Program in Chicago Recommended Citation. *CHILD LEGAL RTS J*. 2014;34. https://lawecommons.luc.edu/cgi/viewcontent.cgi?article=1062&context=clrj

274. CPSTF Finding - Social Determinants of Health: Healthy School Meals for All. www.thecommunityguide.org. Published November 29, 2022.

https://www.thecommunityguide.org/pages/tffrs-social-determinants-health-healthy-school-meals-all.html

275. Shaker Y, Grineski SE, Collins TW, Flores AB. Redlining, racism and food access in US urban cores. *Agriculture and Human Values.* 2022;40(40). doi:https://doi.org/10.1007/s10460-022-10340-3

276. Li M, Yuan F. Historical redlining and food environments: A study of 102 urban areas in the United States. *Health & Place.* 2022;75(1):102775. doi:https://doi.org/10.1016/j.healthplace.2022.102775

277. Linde S, Walker RJ, Campbell J, Egede LE. Historic Residential Redlining and Present-Day Social Determinants of Health, Home Evictions, and Food Insecurity within US Neighborhoods. *Journal of General Internal Medicine.* 2023;38. doi:https://doi.org/10.1007/s11606-023-08258-5

278. Treadway C, Levine A. Why food deserts persist in low-income NYC neighborhoods. PIX11. Published May 17, 2021. https://pix11.com/news/created-equal/why-food-deserts-persist-in-low-income-nyc-neighborhoods/

279. Rhone A, Williams R, Dicken C. Low-Income and Low-Foodstore-Access Census Tracts, 2015–19. www.ers.usda.gov. Published June 2022. https://www.ers.usda.gov/publications/pub-details/?pubid=104157

280. Diet-related cancer burden. NIMHD. https://www.nimhd.nih.gov/news-events/features/community-health/dr_zhang.html

281. Frndak SE. An ecological study of food desert prevalence and 4th grade academic achievement in New York State school districts. *Journal of Public Health Research.* 2014;3(3). doi:https://doi.org/10.4081/jphr.2014.319

282. Dollar Stores Are Targeting Struggling Urban Neighborhoods and Small Towns. One Community Is Showing How to Fight Back. - Institute for Local Self-Reliance. Institute for Local Self-Reliance. Published May 13, 2024. https://ilsr.org/articles/dollar-stores-target-cities-towns-one-fights-back/

283. Odoms-Young A, Brown A, Agurs-Collins T, Karen Glanz RDN. Food Insecurity, Neighborhood Food Environment, and Health Disparities: State of the Science, Research Gaps and Opportunities. *The American Journal of Clinical Nutrition.* 2023;119(3). doi:https://doi.org/10.1016/j.ajcnut.2023.12.019

284. Janczak H. Dying for Groceries: Food Deserts and Mortality Rates in Chicago. Open Works. Published 2016. Accessed December 3, 2024. https://openworks.wooster.edu/independentstudy/10613/

285. Error. www.cdph.ca.gov. https://www.cdph.ca.gov/Programs/CCDPHP/DCDIC/CDCB/CDPH%20Document%20Library/2019%20Diabetes%20Burden%20Report%20(SCOTT_9JUNE2020).pdf

286. Healthy Food Financing Initiative | Rural Development. www.rd.usda.gov. https://www.rd.usda.gov/about-rd/initiatives/healthy-food-financing-initiative

287. KARPYN AE, RISER D, TRACY T, WANG R, SHEN Y. The changing landscape of food deserts. *UNSCN nutrition.* 2019;44:46-53. https://pmc.ncbi.nlm.nih.gov/articles/PMC7299236/

288. Denchak M. Flint Water Crisis: Everything You Need to Know. NRDC. Published October 8, 2024. https://www.nrdc.org/stories/flint-water-crisis-everything-you-need-know#summary

289. Hanna-Attisha M, LaChance J, Sadler RC, Champney Schnepp A. Elevated Blood Lead Levels in Children Associated With the Flint Drinking Water Crisis: A Spatial Analysis of Risk and Public Health Response. *American Journal of Public Health.* 2016;106(2):283-290. doi:https://doi.org/10.2105/ajph.2015.303003

290. *HAZARDOUS AIR POLLUTANTS SPECIAL REPORT.* Accessed December 3, 2024. https://www.houstontx.gov/health/hazardous.pdf

291. Caiazzo F, Ashok A, Waitz IA, Yim SHL, Barrett SRH. Air pollution and early deaths in the United States. Part I: Quantifying the impact of major sectors in 2005. *Atmospheric Environment.* 2013;79:198-208. doi:https://doi.org/10.1016/j.atmosenv.2013.05.081

292. Yao Y, Liu L, Guo G, Zeng Y, Ji JS. Interaction of Sirtuin 1 (SIRT1) candidate longevity gene and particulate matter (PM2.5) on all-cause mortality: a longitudinal cohort study in China. *Environmental Health.* 2021;20(1). doi:https://doi.org/10.1186/s12940-021-00718-x

293. Persico C. How Exposure to Pollution Affects Educational Outcomes and Inequality. Brookings. Published November 20, 2019. https://www.brookings.edu/articles/how-exposure-to-pollution-affects-educational-outcomes-and-inequality/

294. Kalnay E, Kanamitsu M, Kistler R, et al. The NCEP/NCAR 40-Year Reanalysis Project. *Bulletin of the American Meteorological Society.* 1996;77(3):437-472. doi:https://doi.org/10.1175/1520-0477(1996)0772.0.CO;2

295. Reclaiming Their Story: A Reflection on New Orleans' Lower Ninth Ward. Published May 5, 2016. https://projectonfamilyhomelessness.org/2016/05/05/reclaiming-their-story-a-reflection-on-new-orleans-lower-ninth-ward/

296. Knobeloch L, Salna B, Hogan A, Postle J, Anderson H. Blue babies and nitrate-contaminated well water. *Environmental Health Perspectives.* 2000;108(7):675-678. doi:https://doi.org/10.1289/ehp.00108675

297. Clean Up Green Up. Clean Up Green Up. Published 2016. https://cleanupgreenup.wordpress.com/

298. Cool Neighborhoods NYC. NYC Mayor's Office of Climate and Environmental Justice. https://climate.cityofnewyork.us/reports/cool-neighborhoods-nyc/

## Chapter 23

299. Biomarkers of Aging and Relevant Evaluation Techniques: A Comprehensive Review. Aging and Disease. Published

online January 1, 2024.
doi:https://doi.org/10.14336/ad.2023.00808-1

300. Gurkar A. Are you a rapid ager? Biological age is a better health indicator than the number of years you've lived, but it's tricky to measure. The Conversation. Published March 15, 2023. https://theconversation.com/are-you-a-rapid-ager-biological-age-is-a-better-health-indicator-than-the-number-of-years-youve-lived-but-its-tricky-to-measure-198849

301. Hamczyk MR, Nevado RM, Barettino A, Fuster V, Andrés V. Biological Versus Chronological Aging. Journal of the American College of Cardiology. 2020;75(8):919-930. doi:https://doi.org/10.1016/j.jacc.2019.11.062

302. Jung M, Pfeifer GP. Aging and DNA methylation. BMC Biology. 2015;13(1). doi:https://doi.org/10.1186/s12915-015-0118-45.Johnson AA, Akman K, Calimport SRG, Wuttke D, Stolzing A, de Magalhães JP. The Role of DNA Methylation in Aging, Rejuvenation, and Age-Related Disease. Rejuvenation Research. 2012;15(5):483-494. doi:https://doi.org/10.1089/rej.2012.1324

303. Lu AT, Fei Z, Haghani A, et al. Universal DNA methylation age across mammalian tissues. Nature Aging. Published online August 10, 2023. doi:https://doi.org/10.1038/s43587-023-00462-6

304. Topol E. Steve Horvath: Our Epigenetic Age Clocks. Substack.com. Published August 23, 2024. Accessed December 11, 2024.

https://erictopol.substack.com/p/steve-horvath-our-epigenetic-age

305. Galkin F, Mamoshina P, Aliper A, de Magalhães JP, Gladyshev VN, Zhavoronkov A. Biohorology and biomarkers of aging: Current state-of-the-art, challenges and opportunities. Ageing Research Reviews. 2020;60:101050. doi:https://doi.org/10.1016/j.arr.2020.101050

306. Kabacik S, Lowe D, Fransen L, et al. The relationship between epigenetic age and the hallmarks of aging in human cells. Nature Aging. 2022;2(6):484-493. doi:https://doi.org/10.1038/s43587-022-00220-0

307. Zhang Z, Christensen BC, Salas LA. Recalibrate concepts of epigenetic aging clocks in human health. Aging. Published online July 17, 2024. doi:https://doi.org/10.18632/aging.206027

308. Real age versus biological age: the startups revealing how old we really are. the Guardian. Published June 13, 2022. https://www.theguardian.com/science/2022/jun/13/biological-age-startups-why

309. Ying K, Liu H, Tarkhov AE, et al. Causality-enriched epigenetic age uncouples damage and adaptation. Nature Aging. Published online January 19, 2024:1-16. doi:https://doi.org/10.1038/s43587-023-00557-0

310. Bell CG, Lowe R, Adams PD, et al. DNA methylation aging clocks: challenges and recommendations. Genome Biology. 2019;20(1). doi:https://doi.org/10.1186/s13059-019-1824-y

311. Haseltine WA. How Old Are You Really? New "Aging" Clock Provides Clues. Forbes. https://www.forbes.com/sites/williamhaseltine/2024/03/23/how-old-are-you-really-new-aging-clock-provides-clues/. Published March 23, 2024.

312. Topol EJ. The revolution in high-throughput proteomics and AI. Science. 2024;385(6716). doi:https://doi.org/10.1126/science.ads5749

313. Melzer D, Pilling LC, Ferrucci L. The genetics of human ageing. Nature Reviews Genetics. 2019;21(2):88-101. doi:https://doi.org/10.1038/s41576-019-0183-6

314. Morris BJ, Willcox DC, Donlon TA, Willcox BJ. FOXO3: A Major Gene for Human Longevity - A Mini-Review. Gerontology. 2015;61(6):515-525. doi:https://doi.org/10.1159/000375235

315. Miyamoto K, Araki KY, Naka K, et al. Foxo3a is essential for maintenance of the hematopoietic stem cell pool. Cell Stem Cell. 2007;1(1):101-112. doi:https://doi.org/10.1016/j.stem.2007.02.001

316. Zhao Y, Liu YS. Longevity Factor FOXO3: A Key Regulator in Aging-Related Vascular Diseases. Frontiers in Cardiovascular Medicine. 2021;8. doi:https://doi.org/10.3389/fcvm.2021.778674

317. Bernardo VS, Torres FF, da Silva DGH. FoxO3 and oxidative stress: a multifaceted role in cellular adaptation. Journal of Molecular Medicine (Berlin, Germany). 2023;101(1-2):83-99. doi:https://doi.org/10.1007/s00109-022-02281-5

318. Novi Silvia Hardiany, Muhammad, Raya Makarim Penantian, Radiana Dhewayani Antarianto. Effects of fasting on FOXO3 expression as an anti-aging biomarker in the liver. Heliyon. 2023;9(2):e13144-e13144. doi:https://doi.org/10.1016/j.heliyon.2023.e13144

319. Wen D, Gao Y, Wang J, Wang S, Zhong Q, Hou W. Role of muscle FOXO gene in exercise against the skeletal muscle and cardiac age-related defects and mortality caused by high-salt intake in Drosophila. Genes & Nutrition. 2023;18(1). doi:https://doi.org/10.1186/s12263-023-00725-2

320. Jimenez L, Silva A, Giampaolo Calissi, et al. Screening Health-Promoting Compounds for Their Capacity to Induce the Activity of FOXO3. The Journals of Gerontology Series A. 2021;77(8):1485-1493. doi:https://doi.org/10.1093/gerona/glab265

321. Maiese K, Chong ZZ, Shang YC. OutFOXOing disease and disability: the therapeutic potential of targeting FoxO proteins. Trends in Molecular Medicine. 2008;14(5):219-227. doi:https://doi.org/10.1016/j.molmed.2008.03.002

322. Hagenbuchner J, Obsilova V, Kaserer T, et al. Modulating FOXO3 transcriptional activity by small, DBD-binding molecules. Darzacq X, Eisen MB, Francois M, Metcalfe C, eds. eLife. 2019;8:e48876. doi:https://doi.org/10.7554/eLife.48876

323. Apolipoprotein E - an overview | ScienceDirect Topics. www.sciencedirect.com.

https://www.sciencedirect.com/topics/medicine-and-dentistry/apolipoprotein-e

324. Reiman EM, Arboleda-Velasquez JF, Quiroz YT, et al. Exceptionally low likelihood of Alzheimer's dementia in APOE2 homozygotes from a 5,000-person neuropathological study. Nature Communications. 2020;11(1). doi:https://doi.org/10.1038/s41467-019-14279-8

325. Li Z, Shue F, Zhao N, Shinohara M, Bu G. APOE2: protective mechanism and therapeutic implications for Alzheimer's disease. Molecular Neurodegeneration. 2020;15(1). doi:https://doi.org/10.1186/s13024-020-00413-4

326. Mahley RW. Apolipoprotein E: from cardiovascular disease to neurodegenerative disorders. Journal of Molecular Medicine (Berlin, Germany). 2016;94(7):739-746. doi:https://doi.org/10.1007/s00109-016-1427-y

327. Jensson BO, Arnadottir GA, Hildigunnur Katrínardóttir, et al. Actionable Genotypes and Their Association with Life Span in Iceland. The New England Journal of Medicine. 2023;389(19):1741-1752. doi:https://doi.org/10.1056/nejmoa2300792

328. Gornick MC, Ryan KA, Scherer AM, Scott Roberts J, De Vries RG, Uhlmann WR. Interpretations of the Term "Actionable" when Discussing Genetic Test Results: What you Mean Is Not What I Heard. Journal of Genetic Counseling. 2019;28(2):334-342. doi:https://doi.org/10.1007/s10897-018-0289-6

329. Miller DT, Lee K, Abul-Husn NS, et al. ACMG SF v3.2 list for reporting of secondary findings in clinical exome and genome sequencing: A policy statement of the American College of Medical Genetics and Genomics (ACMG). Genetics in Medicine. 2023;25(8):100866-100866. doi:https://doi.org/10.1016/j.gim.2023.100866

330. Halldorsson BV, Eggertsson HP, Moore S, et al. The sequences of 150,119 genomes in the UK Biobank. 2022;607(7920):732-740. doi:https://doi.org/10.1038/s41586-022-04965-x

331. Dewey FE, Murray MF, Overton JD, et al. Distribution and clinical impact of functional variants in 50,726 whole-exome sequences from the DiscovEHR study. Science. 2016;354(6319):aaf6814. doi:https://doi.org/10.1126/science.aaf6814

332. Navar AM, Fine LJ, Ambrosius WT, et al. Earlier treatment in adults with high lifetime risk of cardiovascular diseases: What prevention trials are feasible and could change clinical practice? Report of a National Heart, Lung, and Blood Institute (NHLBI) Workshop. American Journal of Preventive Cardiology. 2022;12:100430. doi:https://doi.org/10.1016/j.ajpc.2022.100430

333. Crosby D, Bhatia S, Brindle KM, et al. Early Detection of Cancer. Science. 2022;375(6586). doi:https://doi.org/10.1126/science.aay9040

334. Haseltine WA. Quantum Leap In Newborn Whole Genome Sequencing. Forbes.

https://www.forbes.com/sites/williamhaseltine/2022/02/08/
quantum-leap-in-newborn-whole-genome-sequencing/.
Published February 8, 2022.

335. The All of Us Research Program Investigators. The "All of Us" Research Program. New England Journal of Medicine. 2019;381(7):668-676. doi:https://doi.org/10.1056/nejmsr1809937

336. Ewart Toland A. New Study Shows the Inaccuracy of At-Home Genetic Tests. Oncology Times. 2021;43(14):15. doi:https://doi.org/10.1097/01.COT.0000767440.84698.b2

337. Gyenis A, Chang J, Demmers JJPG, et al. Genome-wide RNA polymerase stalling shapes the transcriptome during aging. Nature Genetics. Published online January 19, 2023. doi:https://doi.org/10.1038/s41588-022-01279-6

338. Yaqub A, Mens MMJ, Klap JM, et al. Genome-wide profiling of circulatory microRNAs associated with cognition and dementia. Alzheimer's & Dementia. 2022;19(4):1194-1203. doi:https://doi.org/10.1002/alz.12752

339. Stoeger T, Grant RA, McQuattie-Pimentel AC, et al. Aging is associated with a systemic length-associated transcriptome imbalance. Nature Aging. 2022;2(12):1191-1206. doi:https://doi.org/10.1038/s43587-022-00317-6

340. Blood protein signatures change across lifespan. National Institutes of Health (NIH). Published January 6, 2020. https://www.nih.gov/news-events/nih-research-matters/blood-protein-signatures-change-across-lifespan

341. Zubair M, Wang J, Yu Y, et al. Proteomics approaches: A review regarding an importance of proteome analyses in understanding the pathogens and diseases. Frontiers in Veterinary Science. 2022;9. doi:https://doi.org/10.3389/fvets.2022.1079359

342. Moaddel R, Ubaida-Mohien C, Tanaka T, et al. Proteomics in aging research: A roadmap to clinical, translational research. Aging Cell. 2021;20(4). doi:https://doi.org/10.1111/acel.13325

343. Lehallier B, Gate D, Schaum N, et al. Undulating changes in human plasma proteome profiles across the lifespan. Nature medicine. 2019;25(12):1843-1850. doi:https://doi.org/10.1038/s41591-019-0673-2

344. M Austin Argentieri, Xiao S, Bennett D, et al. Proteomic aging clock predicts mortality and risk of common age-related diseases in diverse populations. Nature Medicine. Published online August 8, 2024. doi:https://doi.org/10.1038/s41591-024-03164-7

345. Liu WS, You J, Chen SD, et al. Plasma proteomics identify biomarkers and undulating changes of brain aging. Nature Aging. Published online December 9, 2024. doi:https://doi.org/10.1038/s43587-024-00753-6

346. Serum protein patterns are associated with future diagnosis of Alzheimer's disease. Nature Aging. Published online September 20, 2024. doi:https://doi.org/10.1038/s43587-024-00723-y

347. Rachel, Minta K, Wu LY, et al. Serum Brevican as a Biomarker of Cerebrovascular Disease in an Elderly

Cognitively Impaired Cohort. Biomolecules. 2024;14(1):75-75. doi:https://doi.org/10.3390/biom14010075

348. de Sousa Maciel I, Piironen AK, Afonin AM, et al. Plasma proteomics discovery of mental health risk biomarkers in adolescents. Nature Mental Health. Published online July 31, 2023:1-10. doi:https://doi.org/10.1038/s44220-023-00103-2

349. Lind L, Mohsen Mazidi, Clarke R, Bennett DA, Zheng R. Measured and genetically predicted protein levels and cardiovascular diseases in UK Biobank and China Kadoorie Biobank. Nature Cardiovascular Research. 2024;3(10):1189-1198. doi:https://doi.org/10.1038/s44161-024-00545-6

350. Bredesen D, Amos E, Canick J, et al. Reversal of cognitive decline in Alzheimer's disease. Aging. 2016;8(6):1250-1258. doi:https://doi.org/10.18632/aging.100981

351. Fang W, Chen S, Jin X, Liu S, Cao X, Liu B. Metabolomics in aging research: aging markers from organs. Frontiers in cell and developmental biology. 2023;11. doi:https://doi.org/10.3389/fcell.2023.1198794

352. Rutledge J, Oh H, Wyss-Coray T. Measuring biological age using omics data. Nature Reviews Genetics. Published online June 17, 2022. doi:https://doi.org/10.1038/s41576-022-00511-7

353. Shen X, Wang C, Zhou X, et al. Nonlinear dynamics of multi-omics profiles during human aging. Nature Aging.

Published online August 14, 2024:1-16. doi:https://doi.org/10.1038/s43587-024-00692-2

354. Chen Q, Dwaraka VB, Natàlia Carreras-Gallo, et al. OMICmAge: An integrative multi-omics approach to quantify biological age with electronic medical records. bioRxiv (Cold Spring Harbor Laboratory). Published online October 20, 2023. doi:https://doi.org/10.1101/2023.10.16.562114

355. Wu L, Xie X, Liang T, et al. Integrated Multi-Omics for Novel Aging Biomarkers and Antiaging Targets. Biomolecules. 2022;12(1):39. doi:https://doi.org/10.3390/biom12010039

356. Murata S, Ebeling M, Meyer AC, Schmidt-Mende K, Hammar N, Modig K. Blood biomarker profiles and exceptional longevity: comparison of centenarians and non-centenarians in a 35-year follow-up of the Swedish AMORIS cohort. GeroScience. Published online September 19, 2023. doi:https://doi.org/10.1007/s11357-023-00936-w

357. Partridge L, Deelen J, Slagboom PE. Facing up to the Global Challenges of Ageing. Nature. 2018;561(7721):45-56. doi:https://doi.org/10.1038/s41586-018-0457-8

358. Rezaei A, Bhat SG, Cheng CH, Pignolo RJ, Lu L, Kaufman KR. Age-related changes in gait, balance, and strength parameters: A cross-sectional study. PLoS ONE. 2024;19(10):e0310764-e0310764. doi:https://doi.org/10.1371/journal.pone.0310764

359. Mahmoud Seifallahi, Galvin JE, Behnaz Ghoraani. Curve Walking Reveals More Gait Impairments in Older Adults with Mild Cognitive Impairment than Straight Walking: A Kinect Camera-Based Study. Journal of Alzheimer's disease reports. 2024;8(1):423-435. doi:https://doi.org/10.3233/adr-230149

360. White DK, Neogi T, Nevitt MC, et al. Trajectories of Gait Speed Predict Mortality in Well-Functioning Older Adults: The Health, Aging and Body Composition Study. The Journals of Gerontology Series A: Biological Sciences and Medical Sciences. 2012;68(4):456-464. doi:https://doi.org/10.1093/gerona/gls197

361. Dommershuijsen LJ, Isik BM, Darweesh SKL, van der Geest JN, Ikram MK, Ikram MA. Unravelling the association between gait and mortality - one step at a time. The Journals of Gerontology Series A, Biological Sciences and Medical Sciences. Published online December 6, 2019. doi:https://doi.org/10.1093/gerona/glz282

362. Peterson MD, Collins S, Meier HCS, Brahmsteadt A, Faul JD. Grip strength is inversely associated with DNA methylation age acceleration. Journal of Cachexia, Sarcopenia and Muscle. Published online November 9, 2022. doi:https://doi.org/10.1002/jcsm.13110

363. Bohannon RW. Grip Strength: An Indispensable Biomarker For Older Adults. Clinical Interventions in Aging. 2019;14(1):1681-1691. doi:https://doi.org/10.2147/CIA.S194543

364. LeBrasseur N. Resilience as a Determinant of Healthspan and Lifespan in Mice. Innovation in Aging. 2021;5(Supplement_1):163-163. doi:https://doi.org/10.1093/geroni/igab046.621

365. Cai R, Gao L, Gao C, et al. Circadian disturbances and frailty risk in older adults. Nature Communications. 2023;14(1):7219. doi:https://doi.org/10.1038/s41467-023-42727-z

## Chapter 24

366. Forman DE, Kuchel GA, Newman JC, et al. Impact of Geroscience on Therapeutic Strategies for Older Adults With Cardiovascular Disease. *Journal of the American College of Cardiology.* 2023;82(7):631-647. doi:https://doi.org/10.1016/j.jacc.2023.05.038

367. Kreisberg RA, Kasim S. Cholesterol metabolism and aging. *The American Journal of Medicine.* 1987;82(1):54-60. doi:https://doi.org/10.1016/0002-9343(87)90272-5

368. Carey RM, Moran AE, Whelton PK. Treatment of Hypertension: A Review. *JAMA.* 2022;328(18):1849-1861. doi:https://doi.org/10.1001/jama.2022.19590

369. Chou R, Cantor A, Dana T, et al. Statin Use for the Primary Prevention of Cardiovascular Disease in Adults. *JAMA.* 2022;328(8):754. doi:https://doi.org/10.1001/jama.2022.12138

370. Cooley DA, Frazier OH. The Past 50 Years of Cardiovascular Surgery. *Circulation.* 2000;102(suppl_4). doi:https://doi.org/10.1161/circ.102.suppl_4.iv-87

371. Al-Khatib SM. Cardiac Implantable Electronic Devices. 2024;390(5):442-454. doi:https://doi.org/10.1056/nejmra2308353

372. Song P, Zhao Q, Zou MH. Targeting senescent cells to attenuate cardiovascular disease progression. *Ageing Research Reviews*. 2020;60:101072. doi:https://doi.org/10.1016/j.arr.2020.101072

373. Owens WA, Walaszczyk A, Spyridopoulos I, Dookun E, Richardson GD. Senescence and senolytics in cardiovascular disease: Promise and potential pitfalls. *Mechanisms of Ageing and Development*. 2021;198:111540. doi:https://doi.org/10.1016/j.mad.2021.111540

374. Sweeney M, Cook SA, Gil J. Therapeutic opportunities for senolysis in cardiovascular disease. *The FEBS Journal*. Published online January 25, 2022. doi:https://doi.org/10.1111/febs.16351

375. Suda M, Goro Katsuumi, Tchkonia T, Kirkland JL, Tohru Minamino. Potential Clinical Implications of Senotherapies for Cardiovascular Disease. *Circulation Journal*. 2024;88(3):277-284. doi:https://doi.org/10.1253/circj.cj-23-0657

376. Healey N. Senolytics target cellular senescence — but can they slow aging? *Nature Medicine*. Published online September 2, 2024. doi:https://doi.org/10.1038/d41591-024-00067-5

377. Finch CE. Senolytics and cell senescence: historical and evolutionary perspectives. *Evolution Medicine and Public*

*Health.* 2024;12(1):82-85.
doi:https://doi.org/10.1093/emph/eoae007

378. L'Hôte V, Mann C, Thuret JY. From the divergence of senescent cell fates to mechanisms and selectivity of senolytic drugs. *Open Biology.* 2022;12(9).
doi:https://doi.org/10.1098/rsob.220171

379. Gasek NS, Kuchel GA, Kirkland JL, Xu M. Strategies for targeting senescent cells in human disease. *Nature Aging.* 2021;1(10):870-879. doi:https://doi.org/10.1038/s43587-021-00121-8

380. Lee S, Wang EY, Steinberg AB, Walton CC, Chinta SJ, Andersen JK. A guide to senolytic intervention in neurodegenerative disease. *Mechanisms of Ageing and Development.* 2021;200:111585.
doi:https://doi.org/10.1016/j.mad.2021.111585

381. Wolfram JA, Donahue JK. Gene Therapy to Treat Cardiovascular Disease. *Journal of the American Heart Association.* 2013;2(4).
doi:https://doi.org/10.1161/jaha.113.000119

382. Yuan R, Xin Q, Shi W, et al. Vascular endothelial growth factor gene transfer therapy for coronary artery disease: A systematic review and meta-analysis. *Cardiovascular Therapeutics.* 2018;36(5):e12461.
doi:https://doi.org/10.1111/1755-5922.12461

383. Povsic TJ, Henry TD, Ohman EM. Therapeutic Approaches for the No-Option Refractory Angina Patient. *Circulation: Cardiovascular Interventions.* 2021;14(2).
doi:https://doi.org/10.1161/circinterventions.120.009002

384. Ray KK, Demetris Pillas, Savvas Hadjiphilippou, et al. Premature morbidity and mortality associated with potentially undiagnosed familial hypercholesterolemia in the general population. *American Journal of Preventive Cardiology.* 2023;15:100580-100580. doi:https://doi.org/10.1016/j.ajpc.2023.100580

385. Cattaneo M, Beltrami AP, Thomas AC, et al. The longevity-associated BPIFB4 gene supports cardiac function and vascularization in ageing cardiomyopathy. *Cardiovascular Research.* Published online January 13, 2023. doi:https://doi.org/10.1093/cvr/cvad008

386. Ylä-Herttuala S, Baker AH. Cardiovascular Gene Therapy: Past, Present, and Future. *Molecular Therapy.* 2017;25(5):1095-1106. doi:https://doi.org/10.1016/j.ymthe.2017.03.027

387. Liu N, Olson EN. CRISPR Modeling and Correction of Cardiovascular Disease. *Circulation Research.* 2022;130(12):1827-1850. doi:https://doi.org/10.1161/circresaha.122.320496

388. Carreras A, Luna Simona Pane, Nitsch R, et al. In vivo genome and base editing of a human PCSK9 knock-in hypercholesterolemic mouse model. *BMC Biology.* 2019;17(1). doi:https://doi.org/10.1186/s12915-018-0624-2

389. Sabatine MS. PCSK9 inhibitors: what we know, what we should have understood, and what is to come. *European Heart Journal.* Published online July 23, 2019. doi:https://doi.org/10.1093/eurheartj/ehz514

390. Stein R. For the First time, gene-editing Provides Hints for Lowering Cholesterol. NPR. Published November 12, 2023. https://www.npr.org/sections/health-shots/2023/11/12/1211672034/for-the-first-time-gene-editing-provides-hints-for-lowering-cholesterol

391. Hoekstra M, Miranda Van Eck. Gene Editing for the Treatment of Hypercholesterolemia. *Current Atherosclerosis Reports*. Published online March 18, 2024. doi:https://doi.org/10.1007/s11883-024-01198-3

392. Li T, Yang Y, Qi H, et al. CRISPR/Cas9 therapeutics: Progress and Prospects. *Signal Transduction and Targeted Therapy*. 2023;8(1):1-23. doi:https://doi.org/10.1038/s41392-023-01309-7

393. Zhang ML, Li HB, Jin Y. Application and perspective of CRISPR/Cas9 genome editing technology in human diseases modeling and gene therapy. *Frontiers in genetics*. 2024;15. doi:https://doi.org/10.3389/fgene.2024.1364742

394. National Human Genome Research Institute. What are the Ethical Concerns of Genome Editing? National Human Genome Research Institute. Published August 3, 2017. https://www.genome.gov/about-genomics/policy-issues/Genome-Editing/ethical-concerns

395. Han L, Mich-Basso JD, Li Y, et al. Changes in nuclear pore numbers control nuclear import and stress response of mouse hearts. *Developmental Cell*. 2022;57(20):2397-2411.e9. doi:https://doi.org/10.1016/j.devcel.2022.09.017

396. Yoshida Y, Yamanaka S. Induced Pluripotent Stem Cells 10 Years Later. *Circulation Research*. 2017;120(12):1958-1968. doi:https://doi.org/10.1161/circresaha.117.311080

397. American Heart Association. Stem cell therapy for heart failure reduced major CV events and death, not hospitalization. American Heart Association. Published November 14, 2021. https://newsroom.heart.org/news/stem-cell-therapy-for-heart-failure-reduced-major-cv-events-and-death-not-hospitalization

398. Yamada S, Jozef Bartúnek, Povsic TJ, et al. Cell Therapy Improves Quality-of-Life in Heart Failure: Outcomes From a Phase III Clinical Trial. *Stem Cells Translational Medicine*. Published online November 24, 2023. doi:https://doi.org/10.1093/stcltm/szad078

399. Gulati J, Zhu M, Gilbreth J, Wang S. The Use of Stem Cells in Cardiac Pathologies: A Review. *Georgetown Medical Review*. 2024;7(1). doi:https://doi.org/10.52504/001c.94024

400. Heart Disease. Harvard.edu. Published 2019. https://hsci.harvard.edu/heart-disease-0

401. Tenreiro MF, Louro AF, Alves PM, Serra M. Next generation of heart regenerative therapies: progress and promise of cardiac tissue engineering. *npj Regenerative Medicine*. 2021;6(1):1-17. doi:https://doi.org/10.1038/s41536-021-00140-4

402. Budhathoki S, Graham C, Sethu P, Kannappan R. Engineered Aging Cardiac Tissue Chip Model for

Studying Cardiovascular Disease. *Cells Tissues Organs.* Published online August 6, 2021:1-12. doi:https://doi.org/10.1159/000516954

403. Min S, Kim S, Sim WS, et al. Versatile human cardiac tissues engineered with perfusable heart extracellular microenvironment for biomedical applications. *Nature Communications.* 2024;15(1):2564. doi:https://doi.org/10.1038/s41467-024-46928-y

404. Ajmal L, Ajmal S, Ajmal M, Nawaz G. Organ Regeneration Through Stem Cells and Tissue Engineering. *Cureus.* 2023;15(1). doi:https://doi.org/10.7759/cureus.34336

405. Roodgar M, Suchy FP, Nguyen LH, et al. Chimpanzee and pig-tailed macaque iPSCs: Improved culture and generation of primate cross-species embryos. *Cell Reports.* 2022;40(9):111264. doi:https://doi.org/10.1016/j.celrep.2022.111264

406. Ballard E, Sakurai M, Yu L, et al. Incompatibility in cell adhesion constitutes a barrier to interspecies chimerism. *Cell stem cell.* 2024;31(10):1419-1426.e7. doi:https://doi.org/10.1016/j.stem.2024.07.010

407. Kim MH, Singh YP, Celik N, et al. High-throughput bioprinting of spheroids for scalable tissue fabrication. *Nature Communications.* 2024;15(1). doi:https://doi.org/10.1038/s41467-024-54504-7

# Chapter 25

408. Vincent G, Adachi JD, Schemitsch E, et al. Post-fracture survival in a population-based study of adults aged ≥ 66 years: a call to action at hospital discharge. *JBMR plus.* Published online January 20, 2024. doi:https://doi.org/10.1093/jbmrpl/ziae002

409. Harvard Health Publishing. Preserve your muscle mass - Harvard Health. Harvard Health. Published February 19, 2016. https://www.health.harvard.edu/staying-healthy/preserve-your-muscle-mass

410. Liu D, Wang S, Liu S, Wang Q, Che X, Wu G. Frontiers in sarcopenia: Advancements in diagnostics, molecular mechanisms, and therapeutic strategies. *Molecular Aspects of Medicine.* 2024;97:101270-101270. doi:https://doi.org/10.1016/j.mam.2024.101270

411. Lo JH, U KP, Yiu T, Ong MT, Lee WY. Sarcopenia: Current treatments and new regenerative therapeutic approaches. *Journal of Orthopaedic Translation.* 2020;23:38-52. doi:https://doi.org/10.1016/j.jot.2020.04.002

412. Guerrieri D, Moon HY, van Praag H. Exercise in a Pill: The Latest on Exercise-Mimetics. *Brain Plasticity.* 2017;2(2):153-169. doi:https://doi.org/10.3233/bpl-160043

413. Chow LS, Gerszten RE, Taylor JM, et al. Exerkines in health, resilience and disease. *Nature Reviews Endocrinology.* 2022;18(5):273-289. doi:https://doi.org/10.1038/s41574-022-00641-2

414. Brandauer J, Andersen M, Holti Kellezi, et al. AMP-activated protein kinase controls exercise training- and AICAR-induced increases in SIRT3 and MnSOD. *Frontiers in Physiology.* 2015;6. doi:https://doi.org/10.3389/fphys.2015.00085

415. Affourtit C, Carré JE. Mitochondrial involvement in sarcopenia. *Acta physiologica.* 2024;240(3). doi:https://doi.org/10.1111/apha.14107

416. Migliavacca E, Tay SKH, Patel HP, et al. Mitochondrial oxidative capacity and NAD+ biosynthesis are reduced in human sarcopenia across ethnicities. *Nature Communications.* 2019;10. doi:https://doi.org/10.1038/s41467-019-13694-1

417. Ji Z, Liu GH, Qu J. Mitochondrial sirtuins, metabolism, and aging. *Journal of Genetics and Genomics.* 2022;49(4):287-298. doi:https://doi.org/10.1016/j.jgg.2021.11.005

418. Hicks MR, Saleh KK, Clock B, et al. Regenerating human skeletal muscle forms an emerging niche in vivo to support PAX7 cells. *Nature Cell Biology.* Published online November 2, 2023:1-16. doi:https://doi.org/10.1038/s41556-023-01271-0

419. Tsai SY. Lost in translation: challenges of current pharmacotherapy for sarcopenia. *Trends in Molecular Medicine.* 2024;30(11):1047-1060. doi:https://doi.org/10.1016/j.molmed.2024.05.016

420. Rowe P, Koller A, Sharma S. Physiology, Bone Remodeling. PubMed. Published 2023. https://www.ncbi.nlm.nih.gov/books/NBK499863/

421. Office of the Surgeon General. The Basics of Bone in Health and Disease. Nih.gov. Published 2004. https://www.ncbi.nlm.nih.gov/books/NBK45504/

422. Dimitriou R, Jones E, McGonagle D, Giannoudis PV. Bone regeneration: current concepts and future directions. *BMC Medicine*. 2011;9(1). doi:https://doi.org/10.1186/1741-7015-9-66

423. Remark LH, Leclerc K, Ramsukh M, et al. Loss of Notch signaling in skeletal stem cells enhances bone formation with aging. *Bone Research*. 2023;11(1):1-14. doi:https://doi.org/10.1038/s41413-023-00283-8

424. Sagar Vyavahare, Kumar S, Smith K, et al. Inhibiting MicroRNA-141-3p Improves Musculoskeletal Health in Aged Mice. *Aging and Disease*. 2023;14(6):2303-2303. doi:https://doi.org/10.14336/ad.2023.0310-1

425. World Health Organization. Osteoarthritis. www.who.int. Published July 14, 2023. https://www.who.int/news-room/fact-sheets/detail/osteoarthritis

426. Pereira D, Peleteiro B, Araújo J, Branco J, Santos RA, Ramos E. The effect of osteoarthritis definition on prevalence and incidence estimates: a systematic review. *Osteoarthritis and Cartilage*. 2011;19(11):1270-1285. doi:https://doi.org/10.1016/j.joca.2011.08.009

427. Ng JQ, Jafarov TH, Little CB, et al. Loss of Grem1-lineage chondrogenic progenitor cells causes osteoarthritis. *Nature Communications.* 2023;14(1):6909. doi:https://doi.org/10.1038/s41467-023-42199-1

428. Eckstein F, Hochberg MC, Guehring H, et al. Long-term structural and symptomatic effects of intra-articular sprifermin in patients with knee osteoarthritis: 5-year results from the FORWARD study. *Annals of the Rheumatic Diseases.* 2021;80(8):1062-1069. doi:https://doi.org/10.1136/annrheumdis-2020-219181

429. Song Z, Li Y, Shang C, et al. Sprifermin: Effects on Cartilage Homeostasis and Therapeutic Prospects in Cartilage-Related Diseases. *Frontiers in Cell and Developmental Biology.* 2021;9:786546. doi:https://doi.org/10.3389/fcell.2021.786546

430. Mandal A. What is a Phase 3 Clinical Trial? News-Medical.net. Published January 24, 2014. https://www.news-medical.net/health/What-is-a-Phase-3-Clinical-Trial.aspx

431. AI in Drug Repurposing: Finding New Uses for Existing Medications - Astrix. Astrix Consulting Services for Life Sciences. Published November 22, 2024. Accessed December 23, 2024. https://astrixinc.com/blog/ai-in-drug-repurposing-finding-new-uses-for-existing-medications/

432. Anokian E, Bernett J, Freeman A, et al. Machine Learning and Artificial Intelligence in Drug Repurposing— Challenges and Perspectives. 2024;1(1). doi:https://doi.org/10.58647/drugrepo.24.1.0004

433. Small numbers of sodium channels on cartilage cells have a large effect on joint damage. *Nature.* Published online January 3, 2024. doi:https://doi.org/10.1038/d41586-023-03845-2

## Chapter 26

434. Piccirillo RA. The Lockean Memory Theory of Personal Identity: Definition, Objection, Response. *Inquiries Journal.* 2010;2(08). http://www.inquiriesjournal.com/articles/1683/the-lockean-memory-theory-of-personal-identity-definition-objection-response

435. The Risk and Costs of Severe Cognitive Impairment at Older Ages: Key Findings from our Literature Review and Projection Analyses Research Brief. ASPE. Published January 31, 2021. https://aspe.hhs.gov/reports/risk-costs-severe-cognitive-impairment-older-ages-key-findings-our-literature-review-projection

436. Knights E, Henson RN, Morcom AM, Mitchell DJ, Tsvetanov KA. Neural Evidence of Functional Compensation for Fluid Intelligence in Healthy Ageing. *eLife.* 2024;13. doi:https://doi.org/10.7554/eLife.93327.1

437. McGill University. Office for Science and Society. Published September 29, 2023. Accessed December 23, 2024. https://www.mcgill.ca/oss/article/medical-critical-thinking/if-youre-getting-old-you-can-blame-klotho

438. Cheikhi A, Barchowsky A, Sahu A, et al. Klotho: An Elephant in Aging Research. *The Journals of Gerontology*

*Series A: Biological Sciences and Medical Sciences.*
2019;74(7):1031-1042.
doi:https://doi.org/10.1093/gerona/glz061

439. Vinicius Wanatable Nakao, Caio Henrique Mazucanti, Larissa, et al. Neuroprotective action of α-Klotho against LPS-activated glia conditioned medium in primary neuronal culture. *Scientific Reports.* 2022;12(1). doi:https://doi.org/10.1038/s41598-022-21132-4

440. Dubal Dena B, Yokoyama Jennifer S, Zhu L, et al. Life Extension Factor Klotho Enhances Cognition. *Cell Reports.* 2014;7(4):1065-1076. doi:https://doi.org/10.1016/j.celrep.2014.03.076

441. Castner SA, Gupta S, Wang D, et al. Longevity factor klotho enhances cognition in aged nonhuman primates. Published online July 3, 2023. doi:https://doi.org/10.1038/s43587-023-00441-x

442. Abraham CR, Li A. AGING-SUPPRESSOR KLOTHO: PROSPECTS IN DIAGNOSTICS AND THERAPEUTICS. *Ageing Research Reviews.* Published online October 22, 2022:101766. doi:https://doi.org/10.1016/j.arr.2022.101766

443. Izquierdo JM. Blood platelet factor 4: the elixir of brain rejuvenation. *Molecular Neurodegeneration.* 2024;19(1). doi:https://doi.org/10.1186/s13024-023-00681-w

444. Sidik SM. Older mouse brains rejuvenated by protein found in young blood. *Nature.* Published online August 16, 2023. doi:https://doi.org/10.1038/d41586-023-02563-z

445. A Secret in the Blood: How PF4 Restores Youth to Old Brains | UC San Francisco. www.ucsf.edu. Published August 16, 2023. https://www.ucsf.edu/news/2023/08/425981/secret-blood-how-pf4-restores-youth-old-brains

446. De la Rosa A, Olaso-Gonzalez G, Arc-Chagnaud C, et al. Physical exercise in the prevention and treatment of Alzheimer's disease. *Journal of Sport and Health Science*. 2020;9(5):394-404. doi:https://doi.org/10.1016/j.jshs.2020.01.004

447. Leiter O, Seidemann S, Overall RW, et al. Exercise-Induced Activated Platelets Increase Adult Hippocampal Precursor Proliferation and Promote Neuronal Differentiation. *Stem Cell Reports*. 2019;12(4):667-679. doi:https://doi.org/10.1016/j.stemcr.2019.02.009

448. Leiter O, Brici D, Fletcher SJ, et al. Platelet-derived exerkine CXCL4/platelet factor 4 rejuvenates hippocampal neurogenesis and restores cognitive function in aged mice. *Nature Communications*. 2023;14(1):4375. doi:https://doi.org/10.1038/s41467-023-39873-9

449. Park C, Hahn O, Gupta S, et al. Platelet factors are induced by longevity factor klotho and enhance cognition in young and aging mice. *Nature Aging*. 2023;3(9):1067-1078. doi:https://doi.org/10.1038/s43587-023-00468-0

450. Schroer AB, Ventura P, Sucharov J, et al. Platelet factors attenuate inflammation and rescue cognition in ageing. *Nature*. 2023;620(7976):1071-1079. doi:https://doi.org/10.1038/s41586-023-06436-3

451. A new Alzheimer's drug will cost $26,500 a year. Who will be able to get it? NBC News. https://www.nbcnews.com/health/health-news/new-alzheimers-drug-will-cost-26500-year-will-able-get-rcna64883

452. Chan D, Suk HJ, Jackson BL, et al. Gamma frequency sensory stimulation in mild probable Alzheimer's dementia patients: Results of feasibility and pilot studies. Rajji TK, ed. *PLOS ONE*. 2022;17(12):e0278412. doi:https://doi.org/10.1371/journal.pone.0278412

453. Iaccarino HF, Singer AC, Martorell AJ, et al. Gamma frequency entrainment attenuates amyloid load and modifies microglia. *Nature*. 2016;540(7632):230-235. doi:https://doi.org/10.1038/nature20587

454. Small studies of 40-hertz sensory stimulation confirm safety, suggest Alzheimer's benefits. MIT News | Massachusetts Institute of Technology. https://news.mit.edu/2022/small-studies-40hz-sensory-stimulation-confirm-safety-suggest-alzheimers-benefits-1213

455. Clinical Studies | Cognito Therapeutics. Cognitotx.com. Published 2017. Accessed December 23, 2024. https://www.cognitotx.com/clinical-studies#hope-study

456. Murdock MH, Yang CY, Sun N, et al. Multisensory gamma stimulation promotes glymphatic clearance of amyloid. *Nature*. 2024;627:1-8. doi:https://doi.org/10.1038/s41586-024-07132-6

457. Glymphatic System - Lab Focuses - Nedergaard Lab - University of Rochester Medical Center. www.urmc.rochester.edu. https://www.urmc.rochester.edu/labs/nedergaard/projects/glymphatic-system.aspx

# Chapter 27

## Closing Thoughts

458. Schneider M. With population of aging Americans growing, U.S. median age jumps to nearly 39. PBS NewsHour. Published May 25, 2023. https://www.pbs.org/newshour/nation/with-growing-population-of-aging-americans-u-s-median-age-jumps-to-nearly-39

459. Science X. 65+ age group to outnumber under-15s in Europe by 2024. Phys.org. Published October 11, 2023. https://phys.org/news/2023-10-age-group-outnumber-under-15s-europe.html

460. Scott AJ. The longevity economy. *The Lancet Healthy Longevity*. 2021;2(12):e828-e835. doi:https://doi.org/10.1016/S2666-7568(21)00250-6

461. Chrisafis A. More than 1.2 million march in France over plan to raise pension age to 64. *The Guardian*. https://www.theguardian.com/world/2023/mar/07/nationwide-strikes-in-france-over-plan-to-raise-pension-age-to-64. Published March 7, 2023.

462. Scott AJ. The longevity society. *The Lancet Healthy Longevity*. 2021;2(12):e820-e827. doi:https://doi.org/10.1016/s2666-7568(21)00247-6

463. Megatrends - The Future of Work for the 50+: What does increasing life expectancy mean for the future of work? www.aarpinternational.org. https://www.aarpinternational.org/initiatives/future-of-work/megatrends/longevity

464. Aaron HJ, Schwartz WB. Coping with Methuselah: Public Policy Implications of a Lengthening Human Life Span. Brookings. Published September 2003. Accessed December 23, 2024. https://www.brookings.edu/articles/coping-with-methuselah-public-policy-implications-of-a-lengthening-human-life-span

465. The Immortal : Jorge Luis Borges : Free Download, Borrow, and Streaming : Internet Archive. Internet Archive. Published 2024. Accessed December 23, 2024. https://archive.org/details/jorge-luis-borges-the-immortal

www.ingramcontent.com/pod-product-compliance
Lightning Source LLC
Chambersburg PA
CBHW070759280326
41934CB00012B/2976